M.D. Computing: Benchmark Papers

M.D. Computing: Benchmark Papers

Current Volumes:

Buying Equipment and Programs for Home or Office

Images, Signals and Devices

Tutorials

C. J. McDonald

Editor

TUTORIALS

With 62 Illustrations

Springer-Verlag
New York Berlin Heidelberg
London Paris Tokyo

Clement J. McDonald, M.D.
Indiana University Medical Center
Indianapolis, IN 46202, USA

Library of Congress Cataloging-in-Publication Data
Tutorials / C.J. McDonald, editor.
p. cm.—(M.D. computing. Benchmark papers)
Bibliography: p.
Includes index.
ISBN-13: 978-1-4612-8321-8 e-ISBN-13: 978-1-4612-3726-6
DOI: 10.1007/978-1-4612-3726-6
1. Medicine—Data processing. 2. Computers. 3. Programming (Electronic computers) I. McDonald, Clement Joseph II. Series.
R858.T88 1987
610'.28'5—dc19 87-28464

Softcover reprint of the harcover 1st edition 1988

9 8 7 6 5 4 3 2 1

PREFACE

Ever since the early 1960s, the medical world has awaited the promise of computerization. Many of us were fascinated by the efforts of the pioneers: Homer Warner's computerized diagnosis system, Octo Barnett's medical information system, Howard Bleich's automated acid/base consultant, and Warner Slack's history-taking program were foretastes of what was to come. At first, however, physicians and hospital personnel resisted the computer because it was too slow, too fragile, too awkward, or too costly. But in the late '70s, computerized order-entry systems began to appear throughout hospitals—in clinical laboratories, pharmacies, and even on the wards. The trend toward hospital information systems, which was only a trickle five years ago, is now a steady tide.

Fast, robust, easy-to-use microcomputers are now available for the convenience of individual practitioners in their own offices. Today's office computer provides competent administrative assistance. It handles accounting and payroll functions, speeds the writing of letters and reports, and even verifies spelling and grammar. It can store, locate, and cross-reference journal articles. It will analyze what has been collected, make statistical comparisons, and draw graphs and figures. Microcomputer programs for medical instruction have become common, and a few medical record-keeping programs are now available. Eventually, no matter where they are, physicians will have ready access to computer-stored medical records. Expert assistance in diagnosis and treatment selection will be as close as the nearest telephone, which will provide an immediate link to the office computer.

Since 1983, *M.D. Computing* has explored and explained all of these aspects. Our magazine's major focus is on computer systems that serve the health provider in the home or office environment. *M.D. Computing* has also examined more general computer applications in medical care. Articles about the computer's role in medical imaging, cardiac monitoring, hospital information systems, and artificial intelligence have appeared in its pages.

Our main objectives are to help the health-care professional select and use computer hardware and software, and, more generally, to educate our readers about the rapidly changing field of medical computing. We aim to present practical facts and principles in a probing yet clear and understandable fashion—scientific without being stuffy. The feedback we've been hearing indicates that we have been successful. Flattering comments about *M.D. Computing* have appeared in the editorial pages of the *Annals of Internal Medicine* and the *Bulletin of the Alliance of Continuing Medical Education*. And we are very pleased that the contents of *M.D. Computing* are now listed in *Index Medicus*.

Each issue of *M.D. Computing* contains articles covering a broad range of subject matter and requiring varying levels of technical expertise. A typical issue might contain a review of an office practice management system—of interest to the physician, nurse, and office practice manager. Next to it might be found a detailed article about a language such as *LISP* and how it could be applied to medical problems, or a tutorial about real-time monitoring of a patient's physiological state, along with book reviews and departments reporting on pertinent computer news.

In several cases, a distinct theme has been carried through a series of features in separate issues. To make this information more readily available to our readers, Springer-Verlag is publishing the current line of books, each presenting collected *M.D. Computing* articles on a single theme. Along with articles originally printed in the magazine, each book will include a complete bibliographical index to make the subject more accessible.

The introductory volume, is geared mainly to care providers, especially physicians who are thinking of purchasing computers for their offices. The second book is dedicated to imaging and monitoring—an introduction to computers in bioengineering, which will also serve as a general review of how such systems as CT scanners operate, for the interested health-care provider. The present volume will be of more interest to the novice who wants to know more about how computers work, or who would like to learn some programming skills; all of the *M.D. Computing* tutorials, are included in this volume.

To our knowledge, *M.D. Computing* is the only publication that has systematically reviewed a large number of office practice management systems. These critiques were prepared by a small and knowledgeable corps of objective reviewers. For the current anthologies, we have decided to include some hardware and software reviews when they relate to a particular theme. But product designs are often revised, and the statements in these reviews do not necessarily apply to the *current* versions of the products discussed. The reviews are intended to provide insights into the kinds of criteria that pertain to systems of a given type, and to call attention to possible problems that should be investigated before you purchase a system.

For our regular subscribers, we hope these volumes will provide a convenient way to locate some of the most useful material from past issues of *M.D. Computing*. And for those who want to learn more about a specific area of "computers in medical practice," we hope they will supply most of the information you need.

Clement J. McDonald

Technical note: The articles in this volume were photoproduced from the pages of M.D. COMPUTING. In some cases, adjustments to the original page layouts (or, less frequently, the wording) have been made to accommodate the requirements of a black-and-white anthology, and to permit the removal of purely decorative illustrations.

CONTENTS

Preface v

Understanding Computer Basics 1
Bruce I. Blum

Mainframes, Minis, and Micros: Past, Present, and Future 9
Bruce I. Blum

Bits, Bytes, Words and Numbers 23
Bruce I. Blum

Programming Languages 29
Bruce I. Blum

Computer- Aided Education 37
Ray E. Eberts, Ph.D.

Talk is Getting Cheap 45
Steven M. and Lynn Entine

Selecting A Display Monitor 51
Richard Friedman, M.D.

Presentation Graphics: An Introduction and Review of Four Systems 59
Tull T. Glazener and Clement J. McDonald, M.D.

Putting Doctors Behind Bars 71
Tull T. Glazener and Clement J. McDonald, M.D.

Let Your Computer Do The Talking and The Listening 77
William R. Pearson, Ph.D.

Programming Languages II 87
William R. Pearson, Ph.D.

Programming Languages III 99
William R. Pearson, Ph.D.

Local Area Networks: Why? What? What IF? 105
Donald W. Simborg, M.D.

Talking to Computers in English 115
Alan R. Shapiro

The Current State of Operating Systems: 1983 and 1984 121
Paul G. Truax

An Introduction to Lisp 127
Michael G. Walker and Robert L. Blum, M.D., Ph.D.

Minimycin: A Miniature Rule-Based System 135
Michael G. Walker, Robert L. Blum, M.D., Ph.D., and
Lawrence M. Fagan, M.D., Ph.D.

Index 143

UNDERSTANDING COMPUTER BASICS

BRUCE I. BLUM

Ask 10 people what a computer is, and you will get 10 different answers. But ask those same 10 people how a computer works, and you will get some blank looks. If *you* are not quite sure how your computer works, now is the time to learn. The better you understand your computer, the better you will use it.

DEFINING THE BASICS

The word "computer" comes from the Latin *computare*, meaning "to reckon" or "to figure out." That is what a computer is—a device to help us figure things out, to help us solve problems. As to how a computer works, that is a harder question to answer.

Basically, a computer responds to two types of electrical signals: on or off, true or false. Everything in the computer is represented as series of these on and off signals, each of which is referred to as a BInary digiT, hence the word "bit." A sequence of 8 bits is called a byte. Text characters are represented as special code stored within a byte. Every character (26 upper case letters, 26 lower case letters, 10 numerical digits, 12 punctuation symbols, and a few dozen special characters) has its own unique code—a number between 1 and 128. This standard code is called the American Standard Code for Information Interchange (ASCII). In this code, 7 bits are used to identify the character, and the 8th bit is used as a parity (verification) bit. Parity bits permit internal checking during data transmission. For example, if a code has an odd number of bits in an even parity machine, the parity bit will be set to one and vice versa. When the parity bit is not set as expected, the computer knows that an error has occurred.

ASCII is the standard code used for microcomputers, and almost all peripheral devices (printers and VDTs) accept data transmitted as ASCII characters. Another code, the Extended Binary Coded Decimal Interchange Code (EBCDIC) used in larger computers, employs all 8 bits for the code. It takes 9 bits to record these codes with their parity bit, hence, tape drives for big machines have 9 tracks: one for each bit.

Data, while stored in computer memory, may be stored as either character codes as described above, or in a number of special binary representations. We will describe these representations in another tutorial. Regardless, it is important to know that memory is

BRUCE I. BLUM

Bruce I. Blum has over 20 years experience in developing information systems. He's a member of the Principal Professional Staff of the Johns Hopkins Applied Physics Laboratory and also an Associate Professor of Biomedical Engineering at the School of Medicine.

From 1975 to 1983, Mr. Blum was the director of the Clinical Information Systems Division of the Department of Biomedical Engineering. He was responsible for the design and implementation of major clinical information systems for the Oncology Center and for the Outpatient Department.

Mr. Blum was the Program Chair for the Sixth Annual Symposium on Computer Applications in Medical Care (SCAMC-82), and is the editor of the new Springer-Verlag series Readings in Computers in Medicine. *He received a B.S. from Rutgers University in 1951, an M.A. in History from Columbia University in 1954, and an M.A. in Mathematics from the University of Maryland in 1965. He teaches computer science at the Johns Hopkins School of Engineering.*

CORE MEMORY REQUIRED MECHANICAL ASSEMBLY AND WAS RELATIVELY EXPENSIVE. THAT HAS CHANGED WITH THE ADVENT OF THE SILICON CHIP.

organized as words. Depending upon the machine, a word may consist of 1, 2, or 4 bytes. A word is the largest unit of information that the computer can process within a single cycle. The larger its word size, the faster the computer is. We often refer to machines in terms of the word size of 8, 16, or 32 bit computers.

LOOKING INTO THE CPU

As you can see in Figure 1 everything in the computer passes through the *central processing unit* (CPU). It contains all the logic for such functions as processing instructions, initiating communications with peripheral devices, and managing memory. The CPU has to manage two types of things: the programs (instructions for solving problems) and the data produced (and used) by these programs. It can perform only a few simple instructions, but it does them quickly; it also can put these simple instructions together to produce complex functions.

The CPU contains some special memory words, called *registers*. The computer has instructions to read a word from memory and place it in a register, store a word in a register into memory, and change the contents of a word by adding something to it, shifting its bits around, and so on.

Figure 2 is a more detailed view. Note that it shows four types of registers:

- *Accumulators:* to perform arithmetic and logical functions (two accumulators—register 1 and register 2—are shown in the Figure; the number and types of registers varies with the computer)
- *Program counter:* to tell the address (location) of the next instruction to be executed
- *Data counter:* to hold the address of the data to be processed
- *Instruction register:* to store the CPU's instructions

In general, the application programs only use the accumulators. The other registers are used by the CPU to keep track of what it is to do (the program counter and instruction register) and where it is to get or store data (the data counter).

Besides these registers, the CPU also contains a unit to perform addition, called the *arithmetic logic unit* (ALU). Despite its name, the ALU does more than just add; it also must do shifting, complementing, Boolean logic, and other simple tasks.

To manage all this processing, there must be a *control unit* (CU). It transfers words to and from memory, loads the registers, and interprets the instruction register. It also processes the sequence of basic instructions used to produce more complex operations, such as division and multiplication. In fact, the CU is a computer within a computer. Its instructions are stored as "read only" programs in what is called *microcode*.

The CPU connects to the memory and peripheral interfaces through electrical pathways called *buses*. There is more than one kind of bus. A data bus carries data from the ALU to and from the registers. An external bus communicates between the computer and the peripheral interfaces. There are a number of national standards for external buses, and when people talk about "the" bus, they are generally referring to the external one.

Another integral part of the CPU is the *clock*. It produces regular, periodic voltage pulses that initiate and synchronize all the actions of the CPU. Clock frequency (or *machine time*) is measured in millions of cycles per second called megahertz (MHz). Frequencies for microcomputer systems commonly range from 1–12 MHz. All other things being equal, the faster the cycle time, the better the processing time.

The clock also synchronizes activities throughout the entire computer, therefore, it must be located on the bus that links the memory and interfaces with the CPU.

The CPU contains some of the initial instructions of the computer, but not all of them. Generally, these instructions are in "read only memory" (more about that in a minute). We start the computer by using some fixed code called the *bootstrap*. It does some processing and then sets the program counter so that another set of instructions can continue the processing. The program branches from one set of instructions to another by changing the program counter. Transferring control from the bootstrap to the application programs is one of the functions of the operating system.

How does a CPU process a simple program? Take, for example, the problem of adding A + B and storing the result in C. Three instructions would be given to the CPU as follows:

1. Take the number stored in location A and bring it to the accumulator register.
2. Take the number stored in location B and add it to the contents of the accumulator register.
3. Store the number in the accumulator register in location C.

This is a three line assembly language sequence. To see what the CPU must do to carry out this sequence, we take a detailed look at the internal processing of the first instruction.

We begin with the program counter pointing to the first instruction to be executed: to load the contents of the word at memory address A into the register. The CPU does the following:

1. Gets the word identified by the program counter and loads it into the instruction register
2. Looks at the instruction, which indicates that the address of a word follows
3. Adjusts the program counter to point to the next word of the program

TYPICAL SMALL COMPUTER SYSTEM

Figure 1

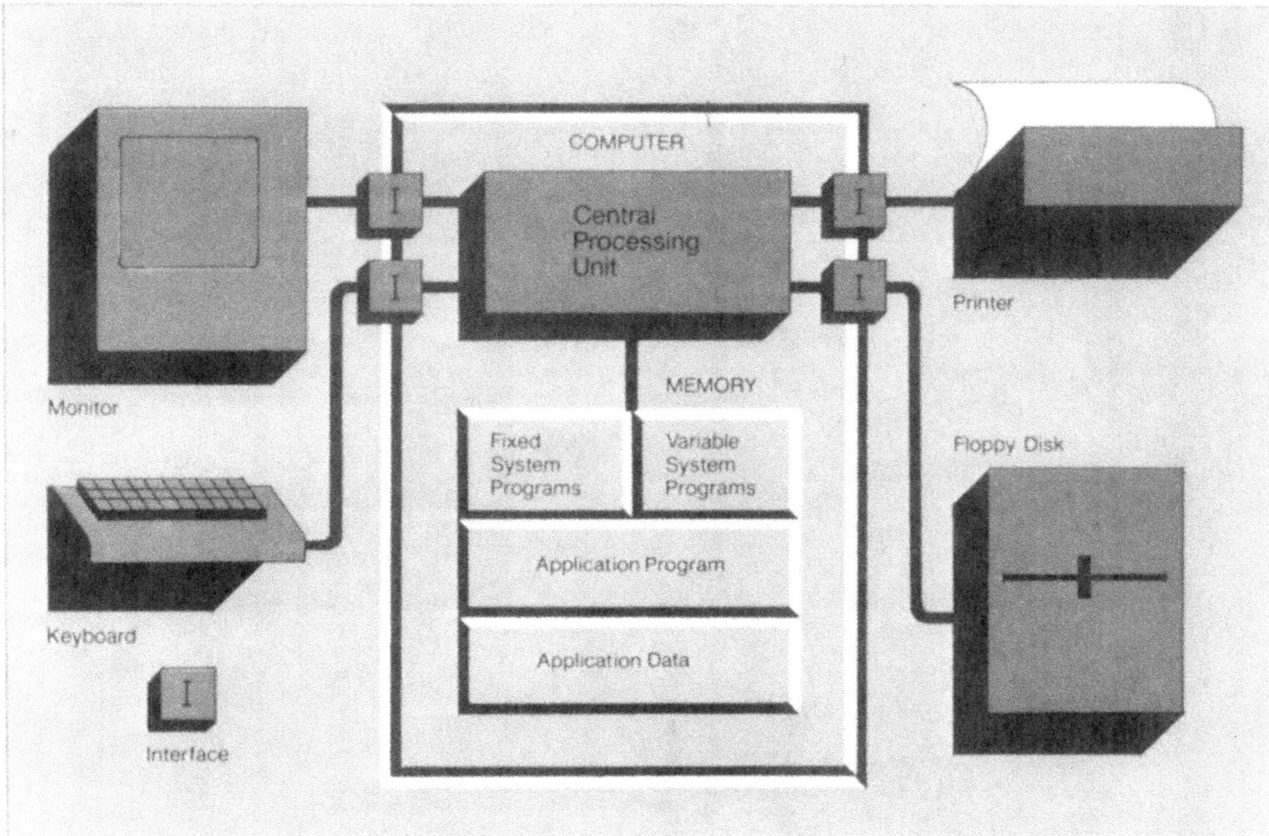

4. Loads this word (the address of A) into the data counter.

5. Starts processing the contents of the instruction register

6. Reads the word whose address is indicated by the data counter and places it in the accumulator register. (If there is more than one accumulator, the instruction has to indicate which one is to be used.)

That is a lot of processing but at 1 million cycles per second it is quickly accomplished.

EXAMINING THE MEMORY

Just below the CPU is a box called the *memory* (see Figure 1). It contains all the information required for processing. When processing is over, the contents of the memory is usually written over or erased. Thus, it is referred to as *working memory*. In Figure 1, the working memory is divided into four sections. The top two contain system programs (fixed memory and variable memory), which are used by the computer to manage the processing of applications. Fixed or *read only memory* (ROM) can be read but not written into (changed). Variable or *random access memory* (RAM) can be both read and written into. Both types of memory are read by supplying the address (the location) of the word desired.

Originally, all computer memory was RAM. The earliest technique was to use tiny doughnuts of magnetic material through which wires were passed. The direction of the magnetism was determined by the electricity flowing through the wires. These doughnut-shaped elements were called *cores* and acted as permanent (nonvolatile) memory for temporal changes in the current. Even today, RAM is commonly referred to as core memory, even though the technology has changed.

Since core memory required mechanical assembly, it was relatively expensive, but that has changed with the advent of the silicon chip that can hold thousands of circuits. These memories represent data as a series of gates, which are either open (conducting) or closed (nonconducting). Today, most memories are comprised of metallic oxide semiconductors (MOS), and are called MOS memories. Unlike core memories, MOS

CENTRAL PROCESSING UNIT

Figure 2

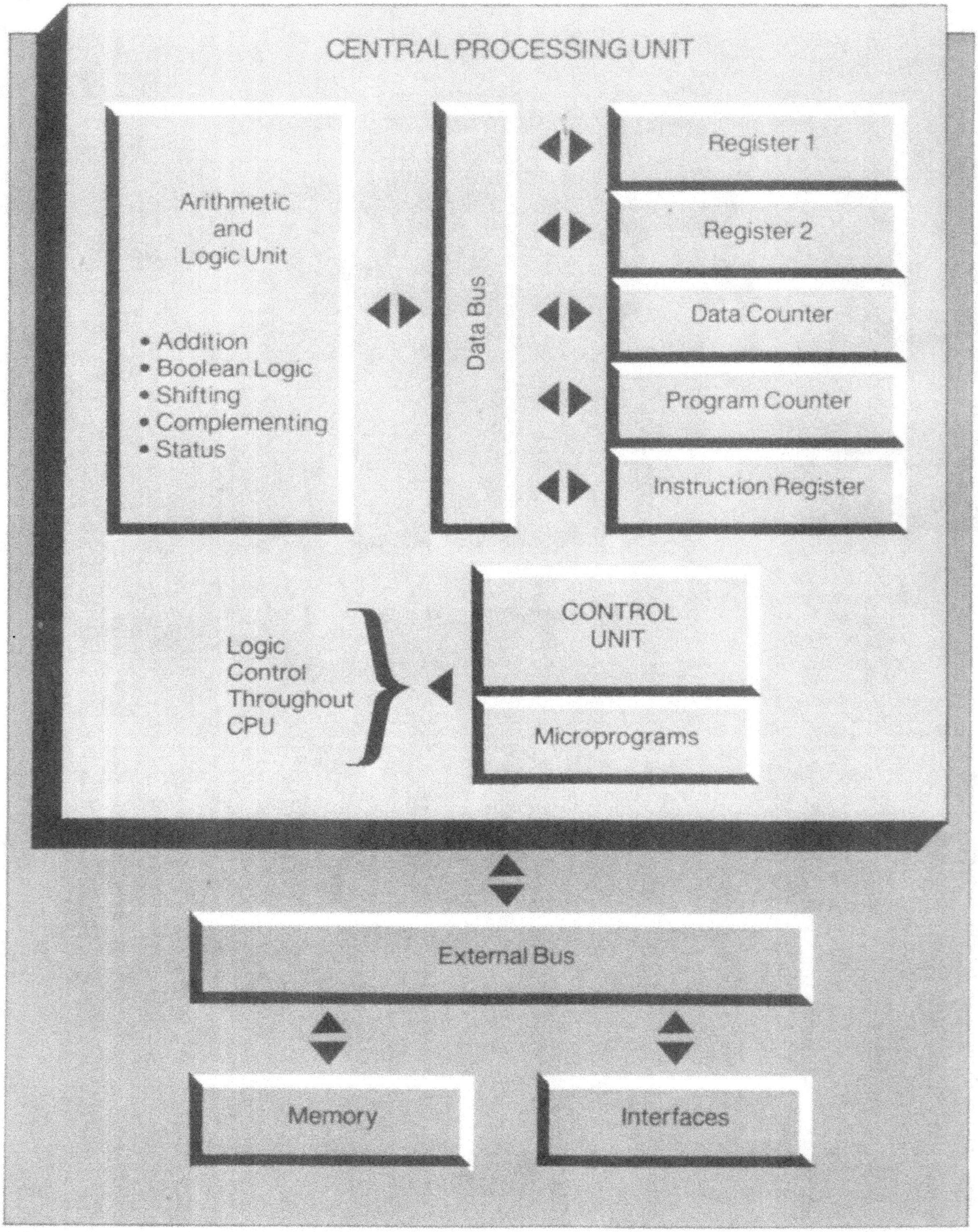

memories lose all their information when the power is turned off, and are therefore said to be volatile. Larger computers normally use backup batteries to prevent loss of the contents of the MOS memory in the event of a power failure. An alternative to MOS is complementary metallic oxide semiconductors (CMOS), which are memories with very low power requirements. They can be powered by flashlight batteries, making them ideal for portable computers.

The advantage of ROM is its permanence; it stores programs that must be available and unchanged. There are several varieties of ROM. The standard ROM is designed for mass production. Programmable read only memory (PROM) is slightly more expensive than the standard ROM but lets you insert your own code. It is best in situations where ROM capabilities are desired, but mass production is inappropriate. Erasable programmable read only memory (EPROM) and electrically alterable programmable read only memory (EAPROM) have all of the permanence of ROM, but also allow writing into the memory under certain circumstances.

COMPUTER JARGON

asynchronous communication	sends one character at a time (used by most microcomputers)
synchronous transmission	sends a continuous stream of characters at one time
bisync	example of a synchronous protocol (set of rules for starting, testing, and stopping transmission)
asynchronous ASCII	transmitting ASCII characters over an asynchronous line
direct memory access (DMA)	the I/O port directly reads or stores data
stealing cycles	when DMA is done parallel with other CPU processing
realtime clock	provides a time reference independent of the computer's clock and can compute the time of day, the time since processing started, or update an I/O buffer for the operating system to read

USING THE PERIPHERALS

The other elements shown in Figure 1 are the monitor and keyboard of the video display terminal, the printer, and the floppy disk. Each is connected to the CPU through an *interface* (a device that defines both the logical and physical connections between the CPU and peripheral devices).

The *keyboard* is your means of communicating with the computer. Each time you depress a key, you send an 8-bit code to the computer. The computer then echoes that code back to a video display; the computer controls what is on the screen. The keyboard sends these 8-bit codes to the computer as fast as you can type.

The number of bits sent to the computer from a peripheral, such as a keyboard, in a fixed period of time is called the *data rate*. It is usually measured as bits of information per second, called *baud*. You can estimate the number of characters sent per second by dividing the send rate by 10. 1200 baud is 120 characters/second.

Video output devices can display full pages (or screens) of output. Since this is done electronically, it can be done very quickly, and the computer can write any character in any position on the terminal. All that is necessary are the commands and circuitry to indicate where and how the character is to be printed, for example, upper or lower case, reverse video, halftone, or blinking. There are no standards for these character placement modes: different terminals use different modes. From the viewpoint of data transmission, however, all character placement commands are just characters to be sent to the output device.

The computer itself does not distinguish between output devices. Sending characters to a video display screen is the same as sending them to a printer. The only difference is that the printer is a mechanical device and cannot process the data as rapidly. Slower printers can operate at 30–45 characters per second. Higher speed printers on small computers can operate at 120–600 lines per minute. Larger computer systems, of course, use faster printing devices. Some nonmechanical laser printers, for example, print thousands of lines per minute.

When sending data to a printer at a high baud rate, control signals are essential so that the printer can signal when it is ready to accept more characters. Where the system needs to transmit characters as fast as the device can print them, a *buffer* (temporary storage unit) is necessary. The buffer may be located in the computer memory, the peripheral, or special interfacing electronics. Characters are sent to the buffer and the printing mechanism reads from it. This eliminates the need to synchronize the sending and printing, as is necessary in some computers.

In some cases, the computer can store more than one line in a buffer; this way, the entire line is listed from the buffer. Some printers list every other line starting from the "back" of the buffer. This allows the printing mechanism to type left to right on one line and right to left on the next. All of this bidirectional logic is in the printer.

OTHER FORMS OF STORAGE

As mentioned before, RAM memory is volatile. This means that when the computer is shut off, the contents of the memory disappears. If all the functions you want to support are already programmed in the ROM, then you have no problem; ROM is not volatile. However, if you want to write programs and keep them available for later use, then you need some way to save the programs when the power is turned off.

The cheapest medium for permanent storage is some kind of magnetic material. It is permanent, erasable, and reusable. Magnetic material is available in several forms; the oldest and least expensive are rolls of tape. Many of the early, low-cost microcomputer systems used tape recorders and tape cassettes as input (I) output (O) devices. Input/output (I/O) was very slow and somewhat unreliable. Duplicating everything compensated for the unreliability, but it made the entire process even slower. The main disadvantage of magnetic tape, however, is that it is a serial device, meaning that you must read through all of the earlier contents of the tape to get at material at the end. You cannot jump around.

The *disk* (or disc) is a flat storage medium that is read and written onto by a unit, which spins the disk and places a magnetic read/write head over any portion of the disk. Unlike the tape, the disk is a *random access device;* you can quickly access any part of it. Disks are available in several forms. The floppy disk is a small (usually 5-1/4 or 8 inches in diameter), flexible disk of magnetic material encased in a protective envelope. The Winchester disk, one type of hard disk, has one or more rigid disks coated with a magnetic surface and mounted in a hermetically sealed container. Still another form of disk allows you to load and unload the disk packs (the recording media) into the disk unit (the read/write device).

The data on the disk are recorded in a series of concentric circles, called *tracks*. Within these tracks, data is broken down into *blocks*. Each block can contain 128, 256, or 512 bytes, depending on the size of the computer.

To read data from a disk, you must first indicate which track you want. There is usually only one read/write head that moves radically from the outer to the inner margin of the disk, track to track. If the disk has more than one surface, these surfaces are mounted on top of one another, like the records in a jukebox. Each surface has its own read/write head, and all the heads move together over the same track. The set of tracks for all surfaces is called a *cylinder.*

By necessity, much of the outer tracks will be left blank. You can tell where a block begins by formating the disk; codes are written out that indicate the location and contents of each block. Disks also have a physical mechanism to provide them with a fixed reference point. In the case of a floppy disk, it is the small hole in the cover near the center. This allow the disk to synchronize as it senses a physical mark. (The format of a hard sectored floppy disk is defined by physical holes in each sector. It comes formatted.)

The speed of a disk depends on how fast the disk spins and how densely recorded the data are. Floppy disks run slowly. The read/write head rests directly on the disk and could damage it if the disk spins too quickly. The capacity of a floppy disk can be increased by using both sides of the disk (double-sided) or adjusting the number of tracks recorded (20, 40, or 80). Double-sided, 80-track floppy disks can store 720,000 characters.

Since hard disks do not let the read/write head touch the surface, they can spin much faster. But hard disks have their problems, too: dust or dirt can scratch the magnetic surface, and the read/write head must be aligned and maintained. As the disk spins faster, the storage density increases, and the tolerance to dust, dirt, and misalignment decreases. Winchester disks have overcome these problems by sealing the unit in a clean chamber and using servos (to control the head position). Since Winchester disks are not removable, they need something to back them up. For smaller units, this means copying to a floppy disk. For larger units a high-speed, dedicated tape unit may be provided.

INTERFACING WITH THE I/O DEVICES

There are two types of I/O interfaces: one for the relatively slow devices, such as keyboards and video displays, and one for faster devices, such as disks. The interfaces receive their signals from the computer's external bus. At the other end, the I/O devices also communicate through interfaces. When these interfaces share the same connections and logic, the computer can communicate to the I/O device.

Interfaces can be serial or parallel. Serial transmission sends one bit at a time (together with control signals); parallel transmission sends one or more bytes at a time. For slower data rates, a serial interface is used; for high data rates, a parallel interface is used. The exception is the printer which can be configured with either a serial or a parallel interface.

Every computer has a fixed number of interfaces for I/O, and each interface is called an *I/O port*. It consists of a buffer and a connection. The transferring of data to or from this device is done by loading or unloading the contents of the buffer. For example, when you depress the keyboard, an 8-bit code is selected, sent across the communication lines one bit at a time, and stored in the I/O port's buffer. When transmission is complete, the computer reads the contents of the buffer to a register, then stores it in RAM, echoes it to the video display, or does whatever the operating system has programmed the computer to do with it.

The peripheral may also have a device of its own for communications and error checking. This is called a *controller* and normally comes on a printed circuit, which can be plugged into the computer's bus.

Control signals govern the communication between the I/O device and the computer. The buffer passes the data. If the CPU does not read the contents of the I/O port's buffer quickly enough, the next input to the buffer will write over the previous input and you will lose data. You can avoid this in smaller computers by constantly examining control (status) bits to see if the transmission is complete. But what if the computer is doing something else when the signal comes in? For this, there is *interrupt I/O* (the ability to interrupt whatever the CPU is doing to pass a message). This is used in multiprocessing systems to signal that an input is ready to be processed or an input is complete. It also interrupts the entire computer to respond to external devices, such as sensors.

QUICK CONCLUSION

This was a very fast tour of how a small computer works. In our next tutorial we will discuss words and their contents. We hope that this article has provided some understanding of the hardware: the CPU, memory and peripherals. We suggest some further reading. We even add a small glossary of jargon you may run into. There certainly is a lot to learn. But fortunately, you really don't have to know too much in order to make effective use of a computer.

SUGGESTED FURTHER READING

Editors of Consumer Guide. *Easy to Understand Guide to Home Computers*. Publications International, Ltd., Signet 1982.

Lieff, J. *How to Buy a Personal Computer Without Anxiety*. Cambridge, Massachusetts: Ballinger Publishing Co., 1982.

Osborne, A. *An Introduction to Microcomputers*. Berkeley, California: McGraw-Hill, Vol. 0, Beginners Book (with David Bunnell), 3rd ed., 1982; Vol. 1, 2nd ed., 1980.

Patterson, David A. *Micro Programming*. Scientific American 248(3):50–57, 1983.

Rinder, R. *A Practical Guide to Small Computers for Business and Professional Use*. New York: Monarch Press, 1981.

Sippl, C., and Mayer, J. *The Essential Computer Dictionary and Speller*. Englewood Cliffs, New Jersey: Prentice-Hall, Inc., 1980.

Toong, Hoo-min D. and Gupta, Amar. *Personal Computers*. Scientific American 247(12):86–107, 1982.

MAINFRAMES, MINIS, AND MICROS: PAST, PRESENT, AND FUTURE

BRUCE I. BLUM

I am old enough to remember when ballpoint pens were first introduced. They were advertised as being able to write under water. The first ones cost fifteen dollars (which was more than an average day's labor in those good old days). I also remember the early digital computers. They were called "giant brains." Ripley's column told me that in order for one to have the power of a human brain, it needed an air conditioner the size of the Empire State Building (which was then the world's tallest building). Well, times change. We know what happened to the ballpoint pen, the value of fifteen dollars, and the relative size of the Empire State Building. They might have been anticipated, but we certainly never expected the computer revolution. In what follows, we shall trace the history of the modern computer, describe how it works, introduce the New Jargon, and project where we are heading. All this in under 6,000 words.

WHAT IS A COMPUTER

There are two types of computers or computing devices. One is called analog, the other is called digital. Both perform measurements and display results. Most computational devices before 1950 were analog. Some examples are watches with a big hand and a little hand, a gas gauge or speedometer on a car, and the tracing of an oscilloscope. In each case, the analog device presents its results as a measure of some mechanical or electrical input which may vary over a continuous range of values. Thus, the automobile's odometer displays the number of miles driven by the mechanical turning of gears. The tenth-of-a-mile unit turns continuously.

Digital devices, on the other hand, perform all their functions in discrete steps. Binary systems, for example, are limited to two elements, "on" or "off" (also named "true" or "false" or, alternatively, "one" or "zero"). In contrast to continuous measures, there is no possibility of a value occurring between the "on" and the "off" of a binary system.

What are the advantages of a discrete system? First, it is very reproducible. If we define a voltage between 4 and 6 V to represent "true", we can be careless in our electronics and still be precise in our calculations. Second, we can convert most information into codes which can be processed discretely. Finally, as we shall see, binary circuits can be mass produced very inexpensively.

SOME EARLY HISTORY

The history of analog computers goes back to Stonehenge and earlier. The use of an analog device for computation may be traced to John Napier, who produced the first book of logarithms in 1640. With this book, one could convert difficult multiplication problems into simpler problems of addition. A computing system—called "Napier's bones"—mechanized this process. Further development yielded the slide rule in 1630. Thus began the happy marriage of engineers and slide rules that lasted until the advent of the hand-held digital calculator.

BLAISE PASCAL

If one ignores the abacus, one can attribute the first digital adding calculator to the philosopher and mathematician Blaise Pascal (1642). Developed to assist him in his work as a tax clerk, the system performed addition through the use of gears. Each digit was separately displayed and a ratchet mechanism was used to "carry" overflows to the next higher digit. Some 30 years later, Leibniz extended the concept to a multiplication machine. However, the concepts were beyond the technology of the time, and these calculators had little practical use.

THE BABBAGE ANALYTIC ENGINE

Charles Babbage (1792–1871) is generally considered to be the father of the programmed computer. Frustrated by the errors he found in the logarithm tables, he sought to develop a machine for making precise computations. Starting in 1822, he began work on a "Difference Engine" which not only computed but also printed the values calculated. Building upon these con-

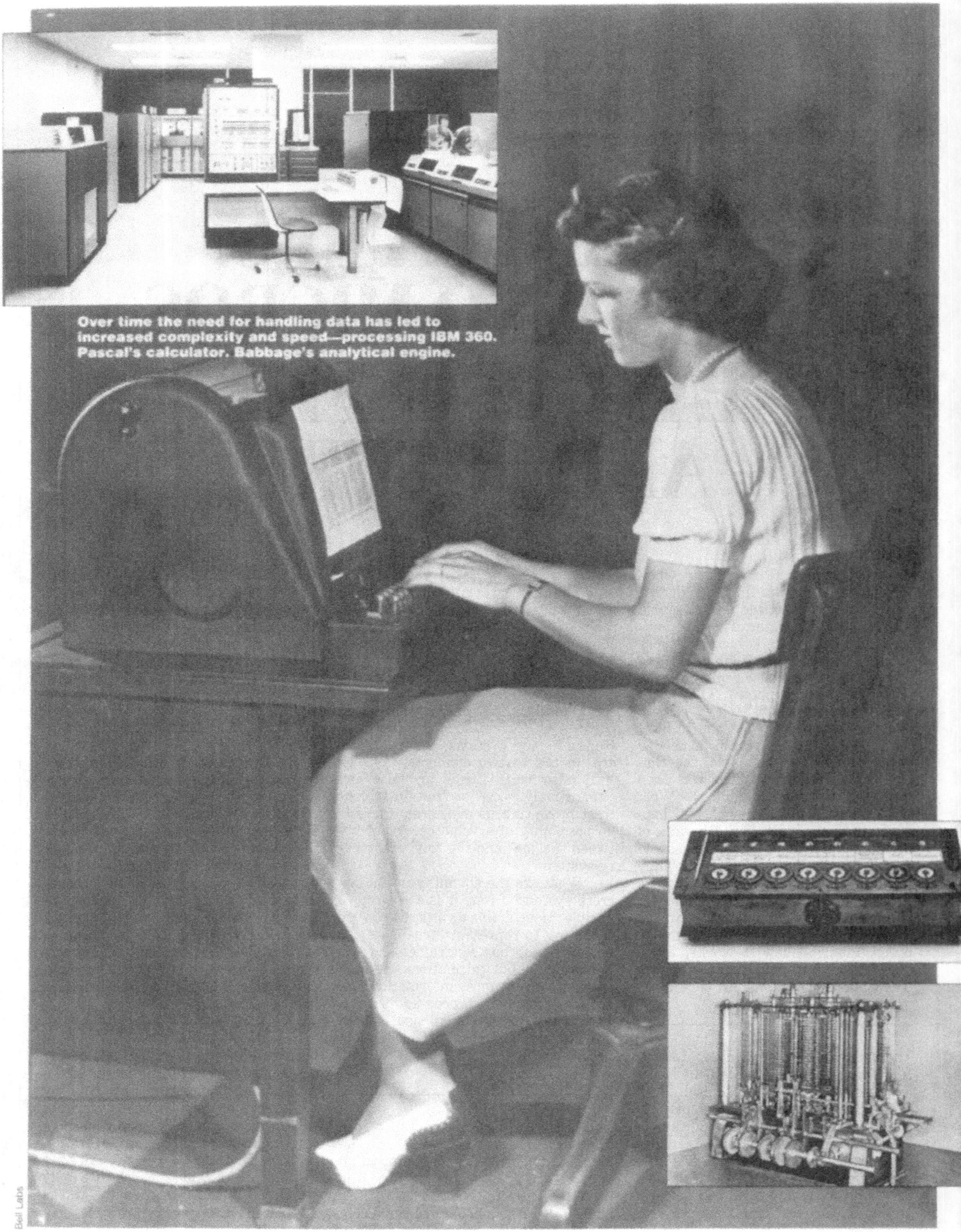

IBM Archive

Over time the need for handling data has led to increased complexity and speed—processing IBM 360. Pascal's calculator. Babbage's analytical engine.

Bell Labs

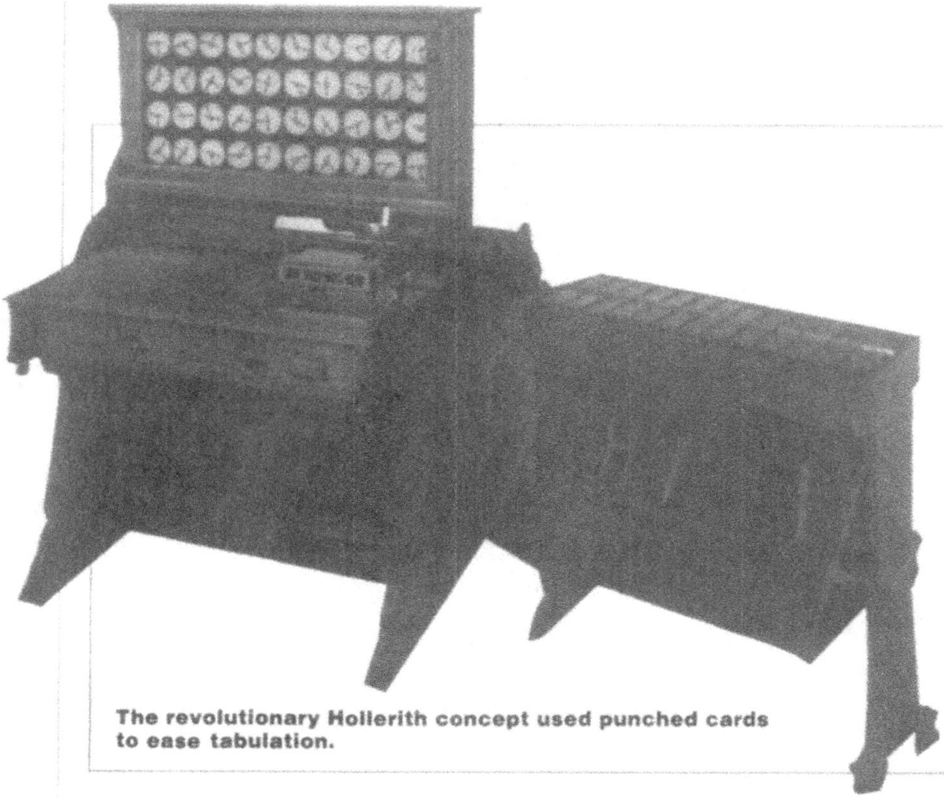

The revolutionary Hollerith concept used punched cards to ease tabulation.

The Computer Museum

cepts, he later turned to the "Analytical Engine" which combined the concepts of computation with stored programs. Copying from the Jacquard loom, Babbage sought to use cards with holes to specify sequences of mathematical commands. As Ada, the Countess of Lovelace and Lord Byron's daughter, put it, "The analytical engine weaves algebraic patterns just as the Jacquard loom weaves flowers and leaves." Unfortunately, a century would pass before a practical operational device was possible.

THE HOLLERITH CARD

The concept of the punch card was developed by Herman Hollerith to manage the 1890 census. The tabulation of the 1880 census had taken seven years, and it was feared that the analysis of the next census would require over a decade. Fortunately, Hollerith began thinking about the problem early and, while on the faculty of MIT, he adapted a punch-card system to meet the special needs of the Census Bureau. The result was a revolution in data processing. In 1896, Hollerith founded the Tabulatory Machine Company which eventually evolved into the International Business Machine Corporation.

THE STIBITZ RELAY-SWITCH COMPUTER

The next fifty years saw advances in mechanical devices for the processing of data in punch-card formats. The time-consuming demands of ballistic table computation led to the development of electronic analog computers in the 1930s and 1940s. In the same time frame, the basic arithmetic circuit, the binary adder, was developed by George Stibitz, as part of his "complex number calculator" (1939). As World War II threatened, interest in these electronic devices grew. Using electromechanical relays to establish the discrete settings, Stibitz and his Bell Laboratory colleagues produced a mechanical computer. It contained 9000 relays, weighed 10 tons and could add two numbers in 0.03 seconds but took an entire second to multiply two numbers. This was the first of a decade of computing machines that performed so well that there was reluctance to invest in the newer electronic devices.

HOWARD AIKEN AND THE MARK I

In parallel with Stibitz's work, Howard Aiken pursued a different vision. His goal was to produce a machine that could output either punched cards or printed material. After three years of work, he discovered Babbage's writing and learned "more about computation from Babbage than any other individual." Aiken began his work at Harvard. In 1939, he received support from IBM and in 1944 installed the Mark 1 "automatic sequence controlled calculator." This contained 3304 relays and 500 miles of wiring. It was slower than Stibitz's machine, requiring 0.3 and 6 seconds, respectively, to add and multiply two numbers, but it was more flexible. A paper tape with holes representing instructions controlled this device and its output could go either to a printer or card punch. It had a productive life of 15 years and spawned the Mark II, Mark III, and Mark IV.

MAUCHLY, ECKERT, AND ENIAC

John Mauchly and J. Presper Eckert took a different approach. They used vacuum tubes rather than electromechanical relays. The advantage was obvious: a vacuum tube could be turned on and off in a millionth of a second. In 1942, they began a four-year development effort that culminated in the delivery of their Electronic Numerical Integrater and Computer (ENIAC) to the Ballistic Research Laboratories in Aberdeen, Maryland. It contained 18,000 vacuum tubes and could perform 5000 additions or 300 multiplications a second. Despite problems of reliability, the computer was used productively for ten years.

JOHN VON NEUMANN'S COMPUTER CONCEPT

Electronic computation had been demonstrated. The next step was the establishment of an intellectual foundation for computing. In 1946, John von Neumann published a classic paper which defined the modern concept of storing the program as well as the data within the computer. Prior to this, instructions were external to the machine and had to be performed in a given sequence or repeated through manual intervention. The use of stored instructions enabled the program to manage processing flow by branching (i.e., the GO TO). Von Neumann worked

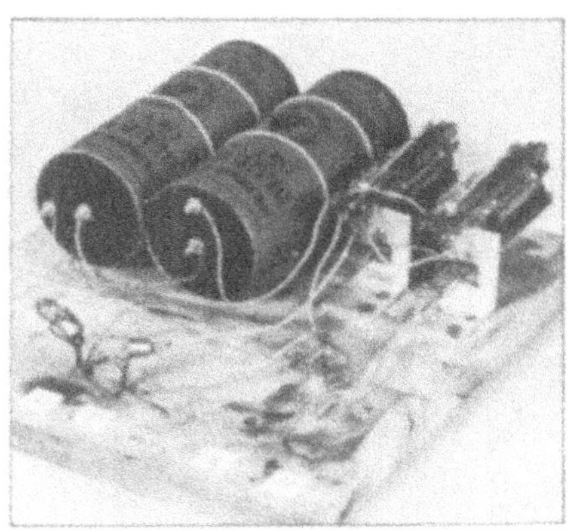

Bell Labs

The Binary adder conceived by Stibitz.

with Eckert and Mauchly to produce the Electronic Discrete Variable Computer (EDVAC) upon which most modern computers are based. For the first time, the binary number system and a stored program were available in an electronic computer. The foundation had been established; improvements in manufacturing technology would bring about a revolution.

THE EARLIEST PROGRAMS WERE WIRED INTO PLUG BOARDS OR PUNCHED ONTO PAPER TAPE.

THE UNIVAC I

In 1947, Eckert and Mauchly left the University of Pennsylvania to form their own company. Their second product was the UNIVersal Automatic Computer (UNIVAC I), which was installed in the Census Bureau in 1951. It contained 5000 vacuum tubes, could add two numbers in 2 microseconds (2 millionths of a second), and employed magnetic tape to speed the input of data. It was the most advanced system of its kind—and remained so for five years.

Financial problems forced Eckert–Mauchly Computer Corporation to sell their company to Remington Rand, who also acquired other leading and complementary engineering firms. These acquisitions provided Remington Rand with early technical superiority over their competitors but did not lead to commercial success. Why?

"From the beginning, the UNIVAC I sales effort was insufficient, unaggressive, and unimaginative. The Eckert–Mauchly personnel, for the most part, had a scientific rather than a business orientation. They realized the limitations of their machine and tended to dampen the enthusiasm of prospective customers who came to them with prophetic visions of the potential of electronic data processing. They knew that these visions would became reality only with a later generation of computers, and they did not encourage the very expensive experimentation which would almost invariably prove them to have been right. Most of this experimentation was eventually carried out on competitor's equipment, spurred on by promises made by salesmen who often understood little or nothing about the capabilities of the equipment they were selling." (Saul Rosen, "Electronic Computers: A Historical Survey," *Computing Surveys*, [1,1] March, 1969)

THE IBM 701

As we know, it was IBM which rose to a position of dominance. We have seen something of their history with punch-card machines and the Mark I calculator. Their product line of the late 1940s included electronic multipliers, an Electronic Calculating Punch, and the Card Programmed Calculator. But it was not until the Korean War stimulated defense spending that IBM announced its first true computer. Delivered in 1953, the Defense Calculator (IBM 701) contained 2048 words of memory and was much faster than the UNIVAC I. As we shall see, good engineering, effective marketing, and a commitment to its customers allowed IBM to grow rapidly from this relatively late start.

TRANSISTORS

Just as the first vacuum-tube computers were being built, the basis for a competitive technology was being developed. While the vacuum tube had great advantages over the relay, its demands for power, dissipation of heat, and limited life all presented problems. The solution was the transistor (for transfer resistor). Developed at Bell Labs in 1947, from semiconducting materials (initially germanium, later silicon), the transistor could serve as an on/off switch. By 1954, the Philco Corporation had developed transistors suitable for use in high speed computers. Thus in 1958, when IBM was ready to introduce the vacuum tube based 709, technology was obsolete.

The transistor ushered in a new generation of computers. Smaller, faster, more reliable; this second-generation computer had a dramatic impact upon the commercial, scientific, and industrial world. Our accomplishments in space exploration, for example, could never have been achieved without them. This was the first wave of the revolution. The number of products and vendors grew too rapidly to catalog them all. Here we shall limit our discussion to one major product: the IBM 7090. In its time, it represented the top of the scientific computer line—it had the computing power of today's home computer.

THE IBM 7090

In 1958, the Ballistic Missile Early Warning System required very fast computers for data analysis and general computation. IBM won the contract by offering to deliver the 709 vacuum-tube computer for program development and promising a transistorized version for operational use. The next year, two 7090s were delivered on schedule. But they were rough prototypes, and scores of engineers went with them to make them work. This shaky start angered IBM users and encouraged competitors. Eventually, however, the bugs were worked out, and hundreds of IBM 7090's (and later 7094's) were sold.

The price of a 7090 was about three million dollars. It contained 32,768 words of memory with each word 36 bits in length. Because both the card-input devices and the printers were relatively slow, each system contained a second, smaller system (generally an IBM 1401 business computer). The smaller system copied the card images onto magnetic tape and/or printed the magnetic tape's contents onto paper. The 7090 "talked" only to the magnetic tape device. (Disk and drum storage devices were not yet commercial products.)

The system, therefore, consisted of a very fast 7090 processor with a bank of magnetic tapes. There was an operator's console with lights to display the contents of important words in the processor's memory. The system completed one job at a time. Computer operators were needed to mount and unmount tapes, and to load cards into card readers. All programs and data had to be punched onto 80 column cards before they could be read into the machine. The computer printer was limited to reports with 120 or 132 characters per line. From these early beginnings, industry standards for computer cards and printers emerged.

PRINTED CIRCUTS

The third generation of computers grew out both a new technology and a desire to correct earlier design limitations. The change in technology came

HARDWARE TERMINOLOGY TREE

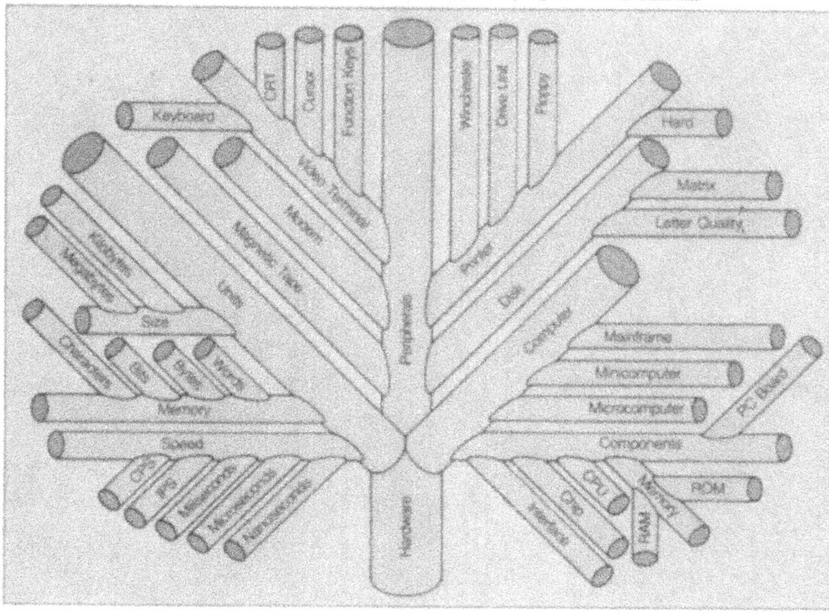

in two steps. First, the use of wires between components was eliminated by printing the connections on a board and then mounting the components to the board. (Thus, the printed circuit.) Then it became possible to etch transistors with their connectors on a chip of silicon. By combining the printing of connections and the etching of transistors, one obtained an integrated circuit (IC). (With advances in manufacturing techniques, the number of components which could be etched on a chip grew. We now speak of large-scale integration, LSI, and very large scale integration, VLSI.)

Lower-cost integrated circuits led to larger and more powerful computers and provided new design opportunities. Second-generation computers typically supported only uppercase letters; it was necessary to change the design of the basic word size and the magnetic tape formats to provide both upper- and lowercase outputs. Second-generation computers addressed either words (e.g., the 7090) or characters (e.g., the 1401). The next-generation machine accessed both. Second-generation computers could process only one job at a time, the next generation, many. A new generation of computers was coming; we had learned so much in so short a time that this new generation would represent a break with the past.

THE THIRD GENERATION: THE IBM 360 SERIES

In 1964, IBM announced their third generation, System/360 computers offered in six compatible models. These computers were intended as replacements for existing IBM computer models but were quite different from them. Consequently, the movement of data and programs from the old machines to the new ones was difficult and costly and customers suffered from the conversion process and resented it. One heritage of this negative experience is that IBM has maintained some degree of compatibility between the System/360 computers and all of its succeeding computer generations. Computer companies with large installed customer bases must evaluate decisions to introduce new technologies by "how they will impact their existing customer base." The reality is that the social investment in computing dampens the rate of technologic change. A corollary to this principle is that the smaller the existing customer base, the bolder the innovation. (And this partly explains the success of microcomputer systems.)

To return to the third-generation computer . . . the problems faced by Eckert and Mauchly were solved. Speed, reliability, and capacity were available. This success led to new and different problems: how were the stored programs of Von Neumann to be managed? As previously noted, the IBM 7090 had 32K words of storage. (In computer jargon, K stands for 1024, which is 2^{10}. Properties of powers of 2 make them convenient units for computers.) The larger computers in the 360 line could contain millions of words of storage (written M for 2^{20} or 1,048,576). Clearly, this was enough storage to hold many programs in memory at once. But this brings up the problem of developing software to manage a computer trying to juggle the execution of many different programs.

SOFTWARE

Hardware is, as its name implies, those parts of a computer system which are composed of manufactured equipment. Hardware is a potential that requires stored programs to actuate. Software is the programs (and associated documentation) which cause the hardware to accomplish a desired goal. The earliest programs were wired into plug boards or punched onto paper tape. As computers grew larger and faster, the programs grew in size and complexity. For small programs, it was sufficient to write the instructions just as they would be processed by the computer. A hole in the paper tape would be a "1," no hole a "0." Certain strings of zero's and one's represented instructions (for example, 001 might be the instruction to add two numbers and 010 might be an instruction to multiply them). A series of such instructions constituted a program. But these were difficult programs to write and debug because the meaning of these instructions was obscured by the codes.

ASSEMBLY LANGUAGE

Better ways had to be found. The first step was to use mnemonics to represent the binary digit (bit) configurations. Thus, if "001" meant "add" to the computer, the programmer could write "ADD" instead of "001" and could use names (e.g., "AVERAGE") to identify the memory locations referenced by his program. The first programming language maintained a one-to-one correspondence between the mnemonic and the machine hardware instructions, but enabled the programmer to use names (or symbols) for the values he wished to process, e.g., X, Y, SPEED. The language was called "assembly language" (or symbolic assembly language) because the process of converting the mnemonic instructions into machine code was called "assembly." Later versions of assembly language allowed the programmer to define a single "instruction" that represented a series of many machine-language instructions. These "larger" instructions are called macros; any assembly language that can accept these is called a macro-assembly language.

HIGH-LEVEL LANGUAGES

Assembly languages provide the most complete control over the hardware and are generally the most efficient. They have serious disadvantages, however. Since the language depends upon the hardware, every computer must have its own unique assembly language. More importantly, because the instructions are very primitive, a great many of them are needed to accomplish a given task. Thus, assembly language programs are prone to errors, difficult to read, and costly to produce. The better way: high-order languages (HOL). For example, if I wish to add three numbers I might think: answer is 10 + 12 + 14. The HOL lets me state this in a natural way.

FORTRAN AND COBOL

The FORmula TRANslator (FORTRAN) allows one to call the answer ANS (or any other convenient name) and use the symbol "=" to mean "compute the value to the right and store (assign) the result in the variable on the left." Thus, ANS = 10 + 12 + 14 is a FORTRAN statement. (Note that "=" does not have the mathematical meaning of equals in the above statement. "ANS = ANS + 1" is a valid FORTRAN statement which means to add one to whatever is in the location called ANS and store this new value back in ANS. It is an invalid mathematical statement since a value can't be equal to itself plus one. Some languages use ":=" as the assignment operator to avoid the misinterpretation that is possible with the "=" sign.)

Starting in the early 1960s, high-order languages such as FORTRAN gained wide acceptance as the best approach to extending the power of the computer. Users were now able to think about their problems in the context of a programming language. Applications which were computational or scientific in nature were written in FORTRAN. As methods for solving problems were developed, the programs were saved in a program library for reuse or exchange. Soon, many of the basic functions were available, and work could progress on more-sophisticated applications. And, in parallel with this, other languages were being developed for other types of applications. The most significant of these, of course, is the COmmon Business-Oriented Language (COBOL). FORTRAN and COBOL represent two of the earliest high-order languages. Each has survived the test of time through continuous modification and a heavy investment in training and program libraries.

SOFTWARE TERMINOLOGY TREE

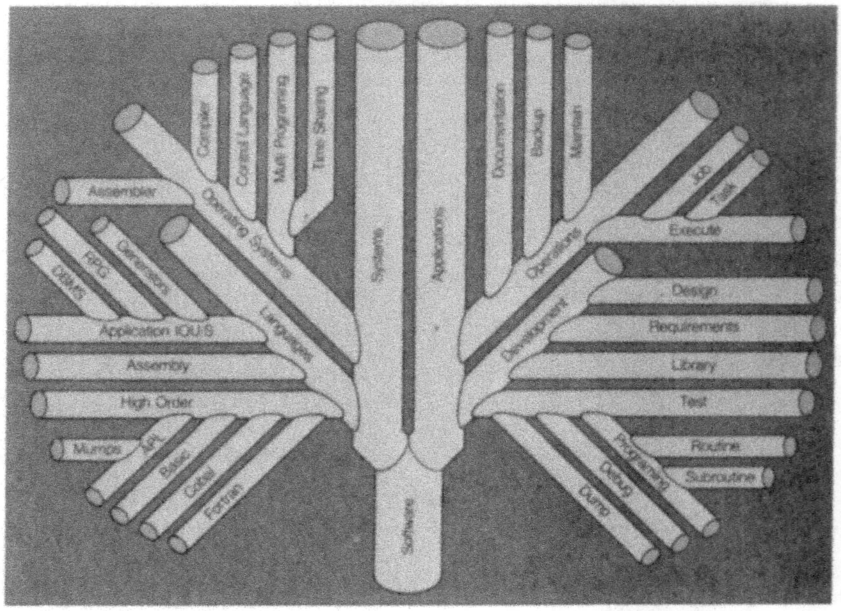

THE OPERATING SYSTEM

As the developers of second-generation computers found ways to improve productivity through high-order languages, they raised a new series of problems.

- The instructions written in assembly language had to be converted to machine code. (The assembler.)
- The instructions written in FORTRAN, for example, had to be converted to machine code. (The process is called compilation and it is done by a compiler. Earlier compilers produced assembly-language outputs for input to an assembler.)
- For some large applications, it was necessary to produce programs composed of more than one separately compiled assembly program. These individual programs had to be linked together and then loaded to run. This was managed by a link loader.
- Application programmers had to provide instructions to inform the computer what they wished done with an application, e.g., run the data for this program, compile the program, or do both. Thus, the need for a command language (or control language or job control language or JCL).
- The input card images on magnetic tape had to be processed, and the material to be listed had to be written onto magnetic tape. Also, the other magnetic tape units had to be managed.
- And when things went wrong? Well, there was nothing else to do but find out why. The standard approach was to list the contents of all the memory locations used by the program. Called a "dump," this listing had a numeric representation of each bit in memory (i.e, the ones and zeros listed in an octal or hexadecimal representation.)

As can be readily seen, that is a lot to manage—even in a second-generation computer where only one job was being processed at a time. Certainly, a tool was needed to manage all of these activities; it was called the operating system.

EVOLUTION OF NEW SYSTEM ARCHITECTURES

Now to return to our chronology. By the early 1960s, we have new manufacturing techniques which allow the production of computers 10,000 times larger than those of the '40s. There are also high-order languages with growing numbers of users who know and care little about the computer's inner workings. And finally, there are experiments with operating systems to bring the users and hardware together. The question is: how can such large machines be used economically? The answer lay in logically dividing one large machine into many smaller ones.

As we have seen, from the days of the UNIVAC I, some computer processes are slower than others. Techniques were constantly employed to avoid slowing down the fastest by off-loading the slowest. Thus, magnetic tapes were used so that the arithmetic processor would not be delayed by the relatively slow card reader or printer. By the time of the third-generation computers, the arithmetic processor had become very fast; so fast, in fact, that even reading a magnetic tape or disk would slow it down. For example, the processor sent a command to the tape to start reading some data. Because the tape has mechanical delays, it could not transmit the data to the processor unit as fast as the processor unit could accept it. And so, thousands of instruction cycles could be wasted while the computer took the time to wind the tape to the location of the desired data and transmit that data to the central processing unit. However, now that the computer memory could contain a million or more words of storage, there was a way to avoid this waste. The computer could keep more than one program in memory at a time. When one program had to get data from magnetic tape, the central processing unit could serve another program that was ready to compute. In this way, computation (i.e., central processing unit, activity) could be balanced with reading and writing (i.e., input and output). On the average, the mix of programs residing in core would complement each other, and the net amount of computer work (throughput) would increase. There was an overhead, of course, that of the operating system needed to manage the whole process.

With the third-generation computers comes a new wave of architectural concepts. There is multiprogramming: the use of a single computer to process more than one job (task) at one time (i.e., to run concurrently). And multiprocessing: the use of more than one central processor unit linked to a single computer system (this redundancy was for graceful failure [fault tolerance] and better throughput). Finally, there was time-sharing (interactive use of a computer using multiprogramming). While the interactive use of computers was explored as early as the late 1950s, it was not until the third-generation computers that it became economical. Time-sharing also was integrated with remote access to a computer which might be miles away, and for the first time users could lease computer time as a utility.

By the mid-1960s, the third generation of computers had been accepted. New applications were proliferating. The new professions of systems analysts and programmers existed. Computers became inexpensive and ubiquitous. Time-sharing allowed users to rent only the computer time they needed. A decade of learning and progress was about to begin.

FOURTH-GENERATION COMPUTERS

We are now using fourth-generation technology. The transition from the third generation is not clearly defined. We know that this is the fourth generation because the Japanese are already at work on the fifth generation—one which goes beyond von Neumann's model. Nevertheless, this is probably a good place to stop in order to review how this computer works. I will, of course, overly simplify.

HARDWARE COMPONENTS

Even if you know nothing about computers to begin with, it now should be clear that it contains "words," a "central processing unit" (CPU), and input/output (I/O) devices. Among the input/output devices are the card reader, the magnetic tape, and the printer. Newer devices include the disk and the video-display tube (VDT, also CRT for cathode-ray tube).

The disk is a rigid platter, coated with magnetic media, similar to that on a magnetic tape. In the case of the disk, several platters normally are mounted on top of one another (much like records in the old-fashioned juke box). The disk spins rapidly and electronic units (heads) are placed just above the surface to read and record information. Because the disks are spinning and the heads are movable, the disk unit can rapidly access information stored in any random location. This is called direct (or random) access; compare it to the serial (or sequential) access method of a magnetic tape, which can require minutes to wind from a datum located at the tapes beginning to one located at its end. A floppy disk is simply a single-disk platter constructed on a soft base and stored in a protective envelope.

The display terminal is both an input and an output device. The keyboard serves as the input. The typical keyboard has at least the standard typewriter keys. It also has extra keys which have special meanings to the computer. For example, when typing with a typewriter, each stroke has an immediate and irreversible action. When typing at a computer keyboard, on the other hand, further action should not be taken until you have completed the input by pressing the RETURN or SEND key. The number of extra keys varies with the terminal; keys beyond the normal set are sometimes called function keys. Some function keys are used to control the cursor. This is a special positioning character on the display screen which indicates where the next character is to be printed. The display screen lists both the inputs to the computer and the outputs from the computer.

ORGANIZATION OF MEMORY

Now we are ready to describe a computer. A simplified diagram is shown at left . The computer contains hardware and software. (The system cannot function without both.) At the top of the figure is the central processing unit (CPU). This is the computer part; it does all the computations. Below it are two storage entities. Working storage (sometimes called main memory or core) is that storage which can be directly linked to (accessed by) the CPU. Everything that the CPU reads, stores, or changes must be in this working storage. All programs which operate in the computer must be in working storage while they run (are executed). All the results of running a program are either printed or transferred to permanent storage (also called mass storage or secondary storage). That is the other reason that we use the name working storage: when the job is completed, everything in it will be destroyed. In this sense, working storage is a scratch pad used by the CPU; when the task is finished, the scratch pad may be discarded.

Since the CPU can only process data in working storage, it is necessary to have some software which can provide instructions on how to do this. This is the operating system. Parts of the operating system are normally fixed into working storage by using read only memory (ROM). These instructions are permanently set at the factory and cannot be modified; i.e., one cannot write on top of the words in a ROM. Other parts of the memory can be both read from and written into. This is random access memory (RAM). In a hand-held calculator, the instructions are all in ROM and only one or two "registers" are in RAM. The keyboard is the input, and there is a one-line output.

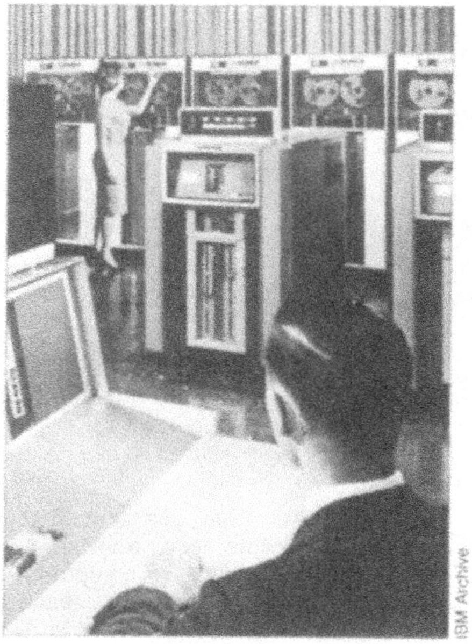

From the vacuum tube to the transistor for processing speed.

The computer shown in the figure is a little more sophisticated. Below the operating system are several "partitions." Each partition (also segment or sector) contains a single program (job, task). This illustrates the multiprogramming concept in which many programs are maintained in working storage with the operating system transferring control from one to another each time an I/O function starts. In most microcomputer systems, there is a single user, and so there is only one partition. In large machines, there may be hundreds of users and associated partitions.

The figure also includes many video-display terminals. Each communicates directly through the operating system to a partition. The program in that partition may be able to respond to the input request, it may have to get some data from the permanent (mass) storage, or it may have to call upon another program to respond to the request. In each of the last cases, the program will request that the operating system get data from the permanent storage. This storage may be disk, floppy disk, tape, or some other storage media. As we pointed out before, everything that will be saved from job to job must be stored on permanent storage. This includes programs and data. Since mass storage is relatively inexpensive, it tends to be much larger than working storage. Access to mass storage, of course, is slower because of its mechanical components.

All fourth-generation computers are modeled after this architecture. The differences are in size, speed, and cost. The microcomputer ranges from the programmable calculator to small multiuser systems; minicomputers are available in single-user configurations or systems which are larger than small mainframe computers. And the mainframes go to large, one-of-a kind processors. The conclusion, therefore, is that labels are becoming less and less useful. Storage is measured in words and "bytes" and speed in microseconds and nanoseconds. But there are few rules for comparing systems. Where a specific application is the goal, the availability or quality of the software may be much more important than equipment size or speed.

THE LAST TEN YEARS AND THE NEXT FEW

In the last paragraph we made some reference to minicomputers and microcomputers. What are they? As you will recall, when integrated circuits were developed in the early 1960s, the third-generation computers were introduced. These were large, multiuser systems which were designed for general-purpose applications. Improved technology resulted in bigger and faster systems. At the same time, there also was an interest in using this new technology to manufacture the equipment of second-generation computers. Such machines, of course, would be smaller and clearly less expensive.

MINICOMPUTERS

The Digital Equipment Corporation was the first to establish itself in this new minicomputer market. Starting with the PDP-5 (1963) and PDP-8 (1965), Digital produced a line of small computers which could become an integral part of some larger system. Initially used as process-control devices or communication managers, the first minicomputers brought the power of digital computers to a new range of products. As part of a larger system, the computer often was embedded in the system's design. Normally, these embedded computers were limited to external sensors to which they had to respond in "real-time," i.e., without delays. Examples of such products and devices include the CAT scanner and military weapon systems. (This use of computers in military systems led to advances in miniaturization and ultimately the microcomputer.)

Although the first minicomputers were used for data collection and processing, it was not long before operating systems were developed and minicomputers became general-purpose, multiuser computers. As manufacturing techniques improved, minicomputers grew more sophisticated while mainframe computers became more compact. By the mid-1970s, the label was meaningless; within the price–performance overlap, there was really no distinction.

MICROCOMPUTERS

The next major breakthrough came when it was recognized that not only could individual circuits be etched in miniature on a silicon chip, but an entire central processing unit (CPU) could be implemented on a chip. In 1971, Ted Hoff of Intel Corporation produced the first "computer on a chip," and now the process went in two directions. Manufacturers, such as Texas Instruments, developed circuits which would have mass markets and produced hand-held calculators, digital watches, and sophisticated toys. Others sought to bring the digital computer to the hobbyists.

The first personal computer, the Altair 8800, was offered in 1975. Selling at $621 (or $395 in kit form), it had limited acceptance and soon disappeared from the marketplace. Those who followed, however, were far more successful. By 1980, some two dozen firms sold 724,000 personal computers at $1.8 billion. The next year there were 20 more firms in the marketplace and the sales were almost $3 billion. A recent study now projects that by 1986, the value of personal computer shipments in the United States will exceed the value of mainframe shipments; they expect 20 million personal computers worldwide with a value of over $67 billion. The big question, of course, is: for what will they be used?

FUTURE TRENDS

And so we have concluded our journey from Stonehenge to the new household appliance. In this brief history, we have focused on three trends. The first—and most dramatic—is the advancement in hardware production. One can expect this to continue with new approaches discovered as we come to the boundary of an existing technology. The second trend is in software. It lags behind hardware by some five years. We are seeing steady improvements in productivity and capability; it is unlikely, however, that software improvements will be as spectacular as those in hardware. Further, because of the low capital outlay required to enter into the software field, it is also doubtful that the quality of software will uniformly approach what we have come to expect in hardware.

The third trend is the application of computers to solving problems. We see computers used in many aspects of our daily lives; from self-banking to supermarket checkout. Word processors are changing the office; electronic mail and public databases are altering our environments. The personal computer (PC) may become an adjunct to our existing communication devices—like the telephone and television; or it may bring changes which we are unable to anticipate.

Although I would not dare to guess what will happen in ten years from now, the trends of the next few years are reasonably clear:

- Just as today's PC's are the equivalent of the second-generation computers, we should soon see the equivalent of third-generation PC's. They will support multiple users, large databases, and full-size displays. One sees these systems now advertised as "professional" systems.
- The distinction between mainframe and personal computers will blur and new architectures will employ networking which integrates the two. Data sources and distributed systems will allow users to merge their personal tools with public resources.
- New classes of peripheral devices will be introduced. These include voice input and output, high-quality graphics, and the marriage of television imaging and personal computing.
- Computer literacy will continue to grow. Younger users will excel in developing new applications; better human factors and engineering will be applied to produce more "friendly" systems.

Each of the above projections is relatively safe, for each is based upon what is available in today's marketplace. The greatest uncertainty lies in the area of how this technology will be applied. By the end of the decade, the tools will be so sophisticated that everyone will be a programmer in the 1970 sense of the word. Unfortunately, these tools are not yet available; consequently today's applications may require an inordinate programming effort, and so the naive owner of a new microcomputer may find it useful, interesting, or frustrating, depending upon his interests and expectations. No matter what his initial impression is, however, he will find it a challenging learning experience which will provide valuable insights into our changing technology.

FOR FURTHER READING

Joseph D. Bronzino. *Computer Applications for Patient Care.* Addison–Wesley Publishing Co., Menlo Park, CA, 1982. There are few texts in the area of medical computer applications. This is highly readable. It contains a historic introduction and chapters on computer applications, including both information systems and embedded computer systems.

Time Magazine. The January 3, 1983, issue made the computer the Machine of the Year. There are some general survey articles, a history, and profiles of some of the major contributors to the microcomputer revolution.

Introductory paperbacks. Most book stores and computer stores have shelves full of introductory texts. Here are three, chosen almost at random, which clearly present the material. There are many others.

Editors of Consumer Guide. *Easy-to-understand Guide to Home Computers.* Publications International, Ltd., 1982, $3.95.

Jonathan D. Lieff, M.D. *How to Buy a Personal Computer Without Anxiety,* Ballinger Publishing Co., Cambridge, MA, 1982.

Robert M. Rinder. *A Practical Guide to Small Computers for Business and Professional Use.* Monarch Press, New York, NY, 1981.

Editor's Note: Coming Tutorials

GLOSSARY

APL (A Programming Language) A high-order language used primarily for interactive mathematical applications. Generally available on larger machines.

Application Software Software designed primarily by users in support of an application. A tool which helps the user in his work.

Application Tools Software systems that provide a desired set of features in a user-friendly manner.

Assembler The system software tool used to translate an assembly language program into processible code.

Assembly Language A programming language in which the language instruction set is very similar to the machine instruction set. Also called symbolic assembly language.

Backup The saving of programs and data in order to retain a recent version in the event of the destruction of the current version.

BASIC (Beginner's All-purpose Symbolic Instruction Code) A high-order language used primarily for interactive programming. Very common on microcomputers.

Bit A binary integer. The smallest unit of information in a digital computer. It takes on the values 1 and 0.

Bug An error in a computer program. Bugs are a natural by-product of programming; they are removed by debugging.

Byte A set of 8 bits used to contain either a binary number or a single character. This is the most common unit measurement for mass storage, e.g., a 5M hard disk has 5M bytes, 5M characters, or $5 \times 1{,}048{,}576 \times 8$ bits.

Central Processing Unit (CPU) That component of a computer in which the computation or processing is performed.

Character Any printable single element such as a letter, digit, or punctuation mark.

Chip A slice of semiconductor material, usually silicon, upon which is printed an integrated circuit.

COBOL (COmmon Business-Oriented Language) A high-order language used primarily for business applications. Very common on larger computers.

Compiler The system software tool used to translate a high-order language program into processible code.

Computer The section of the computer system that contains the processor and memory.

Control Language A system language used to provide information about the job to be run. Sometimes called Job Control Language (JCL).

CPS (Characters Per Second) A measure of printing speed.

CPU See Central Processing Unit.

CRT (Cathode-Ray Tube) A technology used for video terminals and television. Sometimes used as a generic term that includes the keyboard and electronics associated with the tube.

Cursor A special display character on a video terminal that indicates where the next character will be displayed.

Database Management System An application tool that enables the user to define an integrated database and then store, retrieve, and query the database.

DBMS See Data-Base Management System.

Debug To remove errors from a program. Errors are bugs before system release; after that they are defects.

GLOSSARY

Defect A failure on the part of a completed system to perform as specified (advertised).

Development The process in which an initial statement of needs is transformed into a tested, operational application.

Disk A generic name for a storage device in which a thin, flat base is covered with a magnetic media upon which data are stored. The disk spins rapidly and a head reads or writes information from or onto the magnetic media. Any portion of the disk may be read, that is, directly accessed. For different kinds of disks, see hard disk, floppy disk, and Winchester disk.

Disk Drive Unit The unit that contains the disk. In some cases, the disk (or floppy disk) is removable, and the unit is that piece of hardware designed to accept and process the disk.

Documentation Descriptive information about the hardware and software. Includes user manuals, tutorials, reference manuals, and design information.

Dump The listing of the contents of computer memory to show its state at a point where a failure occurred.

Execute To run a task or job.

FORTRAN (FORmula TRANslator) A high order language used primarily for scientific and engineering applications. Very common on larger computers.

Function Keys Special-purpose keys on a keyboard. Each has a special meaning to the hardware or software; none are normally found on a standard typewriter.

Generator A software tool that transposes a set of statements into an executable program. Also called program generator or application generator depending upon the technique used.

Hard Disk A disk made of rigid material as opposed to the plastic base of the floppy disk. Hard disks have more capacity than floppy disks. Frequently, hard disks are configured in stacks, jukebox fashion.

Hardware The equipment that includes the computer and the associated peripherals that comprise the computer system. The hardware does not include the software, which is the set of instructions used to make the hardware perform the desired task.

High-Order Languages (HOL) Programming languages that use application-oriented statements, which describe a function to be performed, e.g., Let X = Y + 2. Contrasted with assembly language.

HOL See High-Order Language.

I/O See Input/Output.

Input/Output Those processing functions that involve input to the computer, e.g., keyboard input, or output from the computer, e.g., printing or writing data to be stored on disk.

Interface Logical: The data passed between two components or modules. Physical: The equipment or standards used to define how data are to be passed between two components.

IPS (Instructions Per Second) A measure of processor speed.

JCL (Job Control Language) See Control Language.

Job One or more tasks to be executed.

GLOSSARY

K Roughly the number 1000; literally, an abbreviation for that power of 2 that is closest to 1000, i.e., 2^{10} or 1024.

Keyboard An input device that is configured like the typical typewriter keyboard.

Kilobytes "Thousands" of bytes where thousands is the power of 2 closest to 1,000, i.e., 2^{10} or K, or 1024.

Letter-Quality Printer A printer in which the individual letters are produced by impact through a ribbon. The most common impact device is called a daisywheel; it has each letter extended on a spoke from a central hub. An alternate configuration is called a thimble; it has the spokes bent into a thimble-shaped configuration.

Library A collection of programs available for re-use in other applications. Also program library.

LSI (Large-Scale Integration) Electronic component parts in which up to 100,000 electrical elements are combined in one chip.

M Roughly, the number 1 million; literally, the power of 2 that is closest to 1,000,000, i.e., 2^{20} or 1,048,576.

Magnetic Tape A media used to store digital information. Data must be read sequentially. Compare with the disk's direct access.

Magnetic Tape Unit A unit interfaced with the computer that reads and processes magnetic tape.

Mainframe Computer A large computer generally costing $250,000 or more.

Maintain The modification of a software system once it becomes operational. This includes removal of defects and the introduction of new functions.

Mass Storage Secondary memory that resides on an external device. Mass storage is used to retain data and programs that are too voluminous to be stored in memory. Data and programs are copied from mass storage to memory in order to be processed, and from memory to mass storage in order to be saved. Mass storage is also called permanent storage; examples are disk, magnetic tape, and floppy disks.

Matrix Printer A printer in which individual letters are made up of individual dots; the printing head moves across the line with pins used to produce the dots that form the letters.

Megabytes "Millions" of bytes where millions is the power of 2 closest to 1,000,000, i.e., 2^{20} or M, or 1,048,576.

Memory The portion of the computer that stores instructions and data for use by the central processing unit (CPU). Sometimes also called working storage. Memory is always accessible by the CPU; contrast this to mass storage, which must be read into memory to be processed.

Microcomputer A small computer using a microprocessor chip. The microcomputer is usually packaged with a keyboard. In personal computer systems, there is generally also a floppy-disk unit and a display. A microcomputer system may offer multiuser support comparable to that of a small minicomputer.

Microsecond A millionth of a second.

Millisecond A thousandth of a second.

Minicomputer A smaller computer generally costing $150,000 or less. Normally multiuser with mass storage.

MODEM (MOdulator-DEModulator) This device is used to link a computer or terminal to and from a telephone line. It converts a digital signal to an audio signal and vice versa.

GLOSSARY

Multiprogramming The organization of a system to enable concurrent execution of more than one separate task. All multiuser systems and time-sharing systems use multiprogramming.

Multiuser System A computer system designed for use by more than one user or task at the same time. Most moderate-to-large interactive systems are multiuser systems.

MUMPS (Massachusetts General Hospital Utility Multiuser Programming System) A high order language used primarily for interactive data-base applications on medium-to-small computers. Started by the medical computing community, many medical applications have been developed in MUMPS.

Nanosecond A billionth of a second.

Operations The use and running of tested, correct programs, applications, and tools.

PASCAL A high order language that combines many of the more-advanced features of block-structured languages. General purpose and powerful, it is available on both large and personal computers.

PC Board (Printed Circuit Board) A board designed to support electronic circuits. Printed circuit implies that some conductive circuits have been applied to the board.

Peripherals The equipment that is used as an adjunct to the computer to produce the final computer system. For example, input/output equipment.

Printer A peripheral used to print output. Microcomputers have available several types of printers, e.g., letter-quality, matrix, and thermal.

Program A collection of instructions that defines the way in which a task should be performed. The program must be translatable into machine instructions that will perform the desired task.

Program Library See Library.

Programming The process of transferring design concepts into a language that can be transformed into machine instructions. The writing of computer programs.

Programming Language A true language that translates knowledge about a task to be performed into instructions that can be processed by a computer.

PROM (Programmable Read Only Memory) Read only memory that will allow programs to be stored through the use of special equipment. The end-user cannot differentiate between PROM and ROM.

RAM (Random Access Memory) Memory that can be both read from and written into. Selection of the word for processing is by address, hence random access. This type of memory is used by programs loaded from mass storage.

Report Generators An application tool that facilitates the preparation of programs that print reports.

Requirements The statement of needs. Tells what a proposed application must do.

ROM (Read Only Memory) Memory that can be read from but not written to. This memory is generally used for system software. The read only property assures that it will not be accidentally destroyed. It is also random access.

Routine An alternate term for program.

RPG See Report Generators; also a specific language for report generation.

Single-User System A computer system designed for use by only one user at a time. Most personal computers are single-user systems.

GLOSSARY

Software The information used by a computer to determine what it should do. By extension, software includes the documentation about this information. Some software (system software) is supplied with the computer equipment; other software (application software) is purchased or developed to meet the needs of a user.

Subroutine An alternate term for program. Implies that it will be used by other programs.

Systems Software Software designed primarily for use by the hardware and the developers of applications.

Task A set of functions to be performed by the execution of a sequence of computer programs.

Test The process by which the developers verify that the product (a) has no errors and (b) performs all the necessary functions correctly.

Text Processor An application tool that facilitates the input, management, and printing of textual information. Compare with word processor.

Thermal Printer A printer in which individual letters are produced as a result of a reaction between a special paper and heat.

Time-Sharing The use of a large, multiprogrammed computer system in which each user typically requires only a small portion of the total resource. Commercially, time-sharing involves the saie of computer resources as a utility.

User One who uses the system. For system software, the user is frequently perceived to be a programmer. For application software the user should be considered a nonprogrammer.

User Friendly A label applied to all software by the seller. In some cases, it is an accurate code word for a support software application that is easy to use and not intimidating.

Video Terminal An output device with a nonpermanent display. Usually a cathode-ray tube (CRT), but other technologies are also used.

VLSI (Very Large Scale Integration) Electronic component parts in which over 100,000 electrical elements are combined in one chip.

Winchester Disk A specific technology for a hard disk. It contains a nonremovable disk unit in a sealed unit. Because of its relatively low price to manufacture, it is the technology generally used for microcomputer hard-disk systems.

Word Processor A fixed system designed to manage the input, modification, and printing of textual information. Compare with the application tool (set of programs) which provides personal computers a text processing capability.

Words A unit of memory that can be directly read. Generally measured in bits or bytes, e.g., 16-bit words.

Working Storage Memory that is used by programs. The information in working storage is discarded at the completion of the job.

BITS, BYTES, WORDS AND NUMBERS

BRUCE I. BLUM

You have heard of 8-bit computers, 16-bit computers, and even 32-bit computers. These numbers refer to the word size. Vendors brag about the "word size" of their computer with phrases such as "a full 16-bit computer." What does this "size" really mean and how does it affect a computer's performance? To answer these questions, you need to know something about a computer's inner workings—how it stores numbers and text, how it does arithmetic, and how it shuttles data and instructions from place to place within its memory. In this tutorial, we will explain these things and thus see how word size affects performance.

By way of review, we distinguish the computer—the hardware that does all the processing—from the peripherals, such as the disk storage, printers, plotters, and the video terminal. The computer itself consists of two major components—the central processing unit (CPU) and the random access memory (RAM)—also called working storage. Within the CPU are a few memory units called registers. These are very high-speed memory devices that play a special role in the CPU. They keep track of details such as the location in memory of the last instruction. They manage the processing of programming loops, e.g., a BASIC FOR loop. They are the focus of most data processing. Data generally must be moved from memory to a register before it can be processed arithmetically or logically.

Between the CPU and the memory is a bus. The bus is the conduit through which all data transfers between the CPU and memory occur. The bus size determines the amount of information that can be transmitted between memory and the CPU registers in one computer cycle. An 8-bit bus can pass 8 bits in one cycle; a 16-bit bus, 16 bits. The register size determines how much information can be processed within the CPU in a single cycle. The word size of a computer is determined by the size of the bus and the size of the general-purpose registers.

With these factors in mind, let us begin our review of the inner workings of a computer by looking at what is called "binary" arithmetic. It is an arithmetic of ones and zeros. First, we will explain how binary numbers and the "text" they symbolize are stored in memory and manipulated by the computer. Finally, we will get back to the question of how word size affects processing speed. The focus of this tutorial may seem narrow, but if you understand these concepts, you will have a better understanding of how your computer works, and also gain insight into how programming languages work.

BRUCE I. BLUM

Bruce I. Blum has over 20 years experience in developing information systems. He's a member of the Principal Professional Staff of the Johns Hopkins Applied Physics Laboratory and also an Associate Professor of Biomedical Engineering at the School of Medicine.

From 1975 to 1983, Mr. Blum was the director of the Clinical Information Systems Division of the Department of Biomedical Engineering. He was responsible for the design and implementation of major clinical information systems for the Oncology Center and for the Outpatient Department.

Mr. Blum was the Program Chair for the Sixth Annual Symposium on Computer Applications in Medical Care (SCAMC-82), and is the editor of the new Springer-Verlag series Readings in Computers in Medicine. *He received a B.S. from Rutgers University in 1951, an M.A. in History from Columbia University in 1954, and an M.A. in Mathematics from the University of Maryland in 1965. He teaches computer science at the Johns Hopkins School of Engineering.*

INFORMATION IS STORED IN COMPUTERS AND MOVES AROUND IN THEM IN DIGITAL FORM AS ZEROS AND ONES, "OFF" AND "ON" ELECTRICAL STATES.

Information is stored in computers and moves around in them in digital form as zeros and ones, "off" and "on" electrical states. Binary arithmetic is the key to this. In fact, computers are binary (two-state) devices. The most familiar arithmetic system is the decimal system which uses ten digits, that is, a base of 10. In the decimal system, every number is expressed as the sum of products of a digit and a power of 10. For example, 3409 is short notation for

$$3\times10^3+4\times10^2+0\times10^1+9\times10^0$$

In decimal arithmetic you add numbers by lining them up according to their powers of 10 and adding their digits, carrying any amount over 9 to the next highest power of 10.

The same procedure is used in any number system, regardless of its base. For example, in the base 2 binary system there are only two digits, one and zero. In any number system, each number is written as a sum of products of digits and powers of the base. Therefore, each binary number is written as a string of ones and zeros. For example, 10101 is the binary number for the decimal number 21. Let us see why. Consider the following: $1 \times 2^4 + 0 \times 2^3 + 1 \times 2^2 + 0 \times 2^1 + 1 \times 2^0 = 10101$; thus 10101 is binary notation for

$$16 + 0 + 4 + 0 + 1 = 21.$$

To avoid confusion, we sometimes write the base as a subscript after the number: $10101_2 = 21_{10}$. With this introduction, there should be no trouble counting to ten in binary.

Decimal	Binary	Sum of Powers of 2
1	1	1
2	10	2 + 0
3	11	2 + 1
4	100	4 + 0 + 0
5	101	4 + 0 + 1
6	110	4 + 2 + 0
7	111	4 + 2 + 1
8	1000	8 + 0 + 0 + 0
9	1001	8 + 0 + 0 + 1
10	1010	8 + 0 + 2 + 0

Adding and Subtracting Binary Numbers

The arithmetic of binary numbers is essentially the same as that of decimal numbers. To add two numbers, you line up the digits according to the base power and add them up from the right. If the sum of any column is greater than an amount that can be expressed with the digits 0 and 1 in base 2 (or 0 through 9 in base 10), then you carry a 1 (or a larger number) to the next highest base power.

Without even concerning yourself with the decimal symbol for the following numbers, you can easily see how they are added:

```
  100101110
 +110011011
 ----------
 1011001001
```

Since long binary numbers are hard to read, the convention is to group the strings of 1s and 0s into series of four, starting from the right. We will do this in the rest of our discussion.

To explain subtraction, we need to borrow the concept of the "additive inverse" from modern algebra. Any number added to its additive inverse equals zero. For example,

$$3 + (-3) = 0.$$

Subtraction is mathematically possible because every number has an additive inverse. In fact, subtraction is really just the addition of an additive inverse. Therefore, the following problems are identical:

Subtraction		*Addition*	
minuend	4	addend	4
subtrahend	2	inverse of subtrahend	−2
difference	2	sum	2

We mention this because inside the CPU is the logic that can quickly add two numbers. In fact, some machines can add two 8-digit numbers in one-millionth of a second, and there are larger machines that can do it even faster. To use this high-speed logic we need, first, to convert subtraction problems into problems of addition. To do this, we need a fast way to compute the additive inverse.

Here is how we do it. First, we form a number called the "ones complement." We do this by converting 1s to 0s and vice versa. Then we add one and call the result the "twos complement." For example, look at the 8-bit numbers below:

0010 0101	number
1101 1010	ones complement
1101 1011	twos complement

Clearly, if you add a number to its twos complement, the sum is a power of two; hence its name. In the example above,

```
  0010 0101 number
 +1101 1011 twos complement
 1 0000 0000 sum as a power of two.
```

Disregard all but the rightmost 8 bits in this example and your answer is, indeed, zero.

Signed Binary Numbers

Keep in mind the positive and negative numbers you learned about in algebra. Normally when we do arithmetic on paper, we use as many digits as required. But the computer divides its memory into fixed-sized units that hold a limited number of bits. (If the numbers you process exceed this limit, the computer quits and gives you an error.) Consider a computer whose unit of processing is 8 bits (also called one *byte*).

In a byte, the decimal number 7 becomes the binary number 0000 0111 and 57 becomes 0011 1001; the twos complement of 7 is 1111 1001 and of 57 is 1100 0111. If you wanted to add −7 or −57, it may be efficient to store the negative numbers in the twos complement form. That is just what many small computers do.

Notice in the example above that the first digit or *leading bit* of the twos complement form is one. For all positive numbers the leading bit is zero. We call this leading bit the "sign bit" because it indicates the sign—positive or negative—of a number. When the computer uses the leading bit to indicate sign, we have only 7 bits left to represent the number's magnitude.

How does the computer know when a leading bit is regarded as a sign bit rather than a bit containing magnitude information in an unsigned number? Your operating system and your application programs keep track of the number type—which is no easy job because, as you will see, there are many different representations for numbers.

Let's look at how the computer multiplies and divides.

Binary Multiplication and Division

Right after you learned addition and subtraction in the third grade, your teacher threw multiplication at you, and long division was lurking in the wings. Well, since binary numbers are all ones and zeros, multiplication turns out to be relatively easy. Again, it follows the same rules used in decimal multiplication. The binary multiplication table, however, is much simpler. Consider the following multiplication problem:

```
    101
  × 101
  -----
    101
   000
  101
  -----
  11001
```

Because we multiply by only ones and zeros, we can convert a multiplication problem into a series of additions. Look at the bits in the multiplier. If the bit is a one, we add the multiplicand to the partial product and shift to the left. If the bit is zero, we simply shift. Since the CPU has logic for shifting as well as adding, that is exactly how the computer does multiplication.

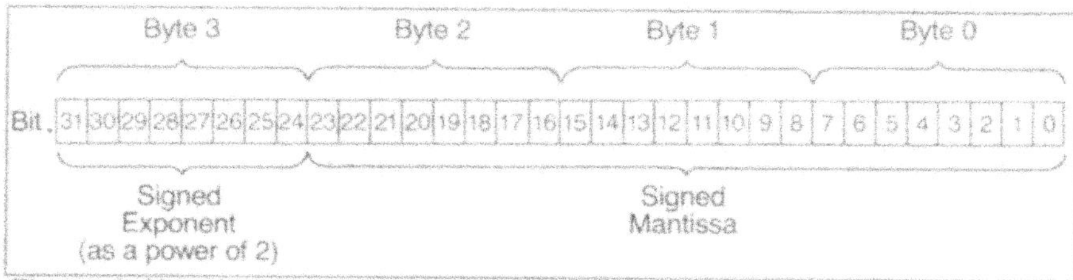

Figure 1. How large numbers are registered within the computer.

What to us is a single operation, to the computer is a sequence of primitive operations. As a result, multiplication is relatively more complicated for the computer—and it takes longer. In fact, the time it takes depends on the number of zeros in the multiplier. The fewer the zeros, the more additions and the longer the processing time. This explains why the speed of some computer instructions varies with the data. Notice that a product may be twice as large (twice as many bits) as either of its multiplicands. To accommodate this reality, the arithmetic register in the CPU is usually twice the computer word size, i.e., a 16-bit computer often has a 32-bit arithmetic register.

Binary division is similar to decimal long division. The computer does binary multiplication by means of a sequence of additions. In an analogous way, it does binary division through a series of subtraction operations. In contrast to the other three arithmetic operations, division creates two answers—the quotient and the remainder.

We have been using 8-bit numbers (or one byte) in our examples to make them easy to read. But a byte does not provide much room for representing numbers. The largest binary number you can record in 8 bits is 1111 1111, which equals *255* in the decimal system—a very small number for most applications. A byte, however, is quite adequate for representing a text character such as an alphabetic letter, a numeric digit, or a punctuation mark. In fact, in most systems text is stored in a sequence of bytes.

CODES FOR CHARACTERS

Did you know that everything that passes to or from the computer begins or ends as characters in some alphabet? Your computer's alphabet contains 26 uppercase and 26 lowercase letters, 10 digits, a dozen punctuation marks, and several dozen special control characters which the hardware recognizes. Each character has a unique code. For exmple, *A*'s code is 65, *5*'s code is 53, and *7*'s code is 55 (see Pearson's article in the January 1984 *M.D. COMPUTING* for the full set of codes). When you type the keys on your terminal labeled "5" and "7" (in that order), the terminal actually sends the code numbers 53 and 55. If the computer has been told to use these 2 codes as a number, it converts them into the binary number 0011 1001, i.e., decimal 57. This is the internal form required to do computer arithmetic, and it has the advantage of compactness. If the computer were to process the "5" and "7" within a word processing document, then it would store the text codes (53 and 55) for those two digits, and the internal result would be:

0 011 0101 0011 0111

—quite different from the previously-mentioned result.

To print the results of a computation, the computer must do the reverse, i.e., convert a binary number into the codes for each digit in the number. Only these codes can be interpreted by your terminal and printer. The fact that a number is represented differently in the computer, depending on whether it is used for computation or for display, can be confusing. However, in a high-level programming language you usually do not have to worry about these conversions since the computer takes care of them automatically.

What would happen if your computer misread one of the bits in the character and sent the wrong code? Obviously, serious errors in the program execution

PROCESSING SEQUENCES

Table 1a Processing sequence in an 8-bit computer.

1. Read the first instruction (LOAD)
2. Read the first byte of the address
3. Read the second byte of the address (CPU now has address of A)
4. Load the first half of A into Register 1
5. Load the second half of A into Register 2
6. Read the next instruction (ADD)
7. Read the first byte of the address
8. Read the second byte of the address (CPU now has address of B)
9. Add the first half of B to Register 1
10. If Register 1 overflows, add 1 to Register 2
11. Add the second half of B to Register 2
12. Read the next instruction (STORE)
13. Read the first byte of the address
14. Read the second byte of the address (CPU now has address of C)
15. Store contents of Register 1 as first half of C
16. Store contents of Register 2 as second half of C

1b Processing sequence in a 16-bit computer.

1. Read the instruction (LOAD)
2. Read the address (CPU now has address of A)
3. Load A to Register 1
4. Read the next instruction (ADD)
5. Read the address (CPU now has address of B)
6. Add B to Register 1
7. Read the next instruction (STORE)
8. Read the address (CPU now has address of C)
9. Store Register 1 in C

could result. To prevent such errors, the computer uses something called *parity bits*. The parity bit is an extra bit which does not carry actual data information; rather it is used as a check on the accuracy of the transmitted data—something like a check digit on a hospital number. The system can be designed for odd or even parity. If the computer was designed for odd parity, the parity bit would be set to 1 if the code contained an even number of "1" bits, and to 0 if it already contained an odd number of "1" bits. In this way, the data taken together with the parity bit would always consist of an odd number of "1" bits. Whenever the computer "detects" a byte with even parity, it knows an error occurred. The parity bit is particularly useful since even a speck of dust on a magnetic disk could cause an error. When the software system detects an error, it tries to reread (rewrite) the character a few times. If it keeps reading errors, it aborts the run.

Using one bit for parity makes the character string longer. But this is not a problem because most computer "alphabets" have only 128 different codes, and 128 codes can be expressed in 7 bits. So the eighth bit can be used as the parity bit. The American Standard Code for Information Interchange (ASCII) is used by all microcomputer applications. Each code is written in 7 bits. For example, 100 0001 is the symbol for the character *A*, 110 0001 stands for *a*, and 100 0010 stands for *B*.

IBM provides another standard 8-bit code called EBCDIC (Extended Binary Coded Decimal Interchange Code) for its large computers, and an extended ASCII code for its personal computer. In the latter, there are 256 different characters, including musical notes and even a smiley face. Since the 256 codes require all 8 bits of the byte, the hardware supplies the parity bit.

Word size is not as important to applications that process only text. Such applications typically process one character (8 bits) at a time. Thus, many successful word processing systems are built upon 8-bit computers. However, 16-bit computers have some advantage, even for processing text, as we will see below.

REPRESENTING LARGE NUMBERS

Now you should understand why the byte is not ordinarily used to represent numbers within the computer. The largest number you can fit into 8 bits is 1111 1111, the number 255. If the first bit is used as a sign bit, then the range of numbers is only from −127 to 127. Obviously, these numbers are too small for most practical applications. Let's see how to represent numbers as large as 10^{38}.

One approach for storing larger numbers is to dedicate two consecutive bytes in the computer to each number. You can fit a positive number as large as $2^{16}-1$ or 65,535 in 16 bits. That is one less than the number that we refer to in computerese as "64K" because it is 64 × 1024; and it is a number large enough for many microcomputer applications. Generally, it is called an integer, and the 16 bits are called the *integer format*. A 16-bit computer has the advantage that it can add two of these integers in a single computer cycle. An 8-bit computer might require 10 or 20 cycles to add the same two numbers because it has to break the problems into smaller steps that fit into 8-bit sizes.

Some problems require even larger numbers. For these, we can use four consecutive bytes (32 bits) as a unit. A 32-bit unit can hold a number as large as 4 billion. Obviously, 32-bit computers would have a speed advantage in doing arithmetic on really large numbers. Still there is the problem of representing fractions like 1.98, 3.14, or 2/3. There are two ways to manage this: the first is called "scaling the integers;" the second is to use scientific notation.

In scaling the integers, we use the binary equivalent of a decimal point. For example, in decimal arithmetic we normally convert the fraction to a decimal approximation. Thus, 2/3 becomes .6667. To add fractions, we line up the "decimal points" and apply the normal addition algorithm. For a computer to do this, it would have to have a "binary point." Since there is no way to designate the binary point within a binary number, the software must keep track of the binary point's location. In other words, the program must know how the number is scaled.

Scaling is a common technique in applications where processing speed is critical. Yet, the use of this technique requires great care to avoid improper changes in scale. The use of floating point arithmetic offers a safer and more flexible technique.

FLOATING POINT ARITHMETIC

Scientific notation represents numbers as the product of a value and a power of 10. For example:

$$.32 \times 10^{-4}$$
$$.765332 \times 10^{12}$$

We can adopt a similar notation (in binary form) to store a number in four bytes. One byte represents the signed exponent (as a power of 2) and the remaining three bytes contain the signed value. The former is called the "exponent" or "characteristic;" the latter is called the "mantissa." If we follow convention by numbering the bits from right to left, starting at zero, the bytes which represent a given number look like the figure on page 25.

Multiplication (division) involves adding (subtracting) the exponents, multiplying (dividing) the mantissas, and adjusting the exponents by removing leading zeros in the mantissa. Addition and subtraction are done by shifting one mantissa to get identical exponents, and then adding or subtracting. Obviously, floating point arithmetic is more complicated (and slower) than integer arithmetic. With floating point numbers

IF THE NUMBER OF PROCESSING CYCLES PER SECOND IS CONSTANT, THEN A 16-BIT COMPUTER WILL BE FASTER THAN ITS 8-BIT COUNTERPART.

that use four bytes, the absolute values range from $.29 \times 10^{-38}$ to $.17 \times 10^{39}$. This is one of the most flexible ways to represent numbers, and it is essential for scientific calculations. But one pays a price for it.

Remember that the CPU handles all this with many small, primitive steps. An 8-bit machine will use its adding logic to add 8-bit numbers. To multiply 8-bit numbers, it will use its shifting and adding logic. Therefore, the 8-bit machine must use more than one step to add numbers stored as 16-bit numbers. The situation is even worse with floating point arithmetic, which takes 50–100 times as much processing time as integer arithmetic. Thus flexibility is achieved at the cost of processing time. Fortunately, many computers support floating point hardware which provides special logic to speed up computations of this kind.

BYTES AND WORDS

We have just seen how a computer represents information. In one byte we can store

- A single character (or code)
- A small number (up to 255)

In two bytes we can store

- A signed integer (−32,767 to 32,767)
- A scaled number (16 bits of information)

In four bits we can store

- A floating point number (absolute range of $.29 \times 10^{-38}$ to $.17 \times 10^{39}$)

And there are data formats that require even more bytes.

The size of the byte is the same in every machine. It is always 8 bits. A word is the largest number of bits that the computer can process as a single unit. In a 16-bit computer, a word is 16 bits. In a 32-bit computer, it is 32 bits. High-level languages can process units that are larger than the computer's word size, but at a high cost in computer time since the computer simulates operations on larger units by performing many steps on word-sized units.

PROGRAM STORAGE

We have already seen how data can be stored in words. Now we consider (in an oversimplified way) the storage of programs. Programs are made up of instructions to the CPU. As we discussed in the previous issue, the instructions tell the CPU what to do with a CPU register and/or a single word in memory. This means that one form for a program instruction is made up of 2 parts: a code to indicate what the CPU is to do and the address of a word for the CPU to use.

As an example, let us add the number which is stored in the word whose address is A to the number stored in the word with the address B and store the sum in the word with the address C. (A, B, and C are symbols for the actual address which is a number. We use the symbols because they are easier to write. Address A actually might be be 0100 0111 1001 0011.)

To have the computer store C as A + B, it might have to go through the following sequence:

- LOAD the contents of word A into register 1.
- ADD the contents of word B to the contents of register 1.
- STORE the contents of register 1 in word C.

This could be written as an assembly language program as follows:

```
■ LOAD    A
■ ADD     B
■ STORE   C
```

The code for each instruction (LOAD, ADD, STORE) can be represented as a 1-byte code to the CPU. The address for each instruction (A, B, C) requires two bytes. Thus, in this case, each instruction requires three bytes, and the program requires a total of nine bytes for instructions. (Not all instructions require three bytes. The instruction to STOP uses only one.)

So far we have seen two advantages of larger word-size computers over smaller ones. The larger the word size, the faster the computer can perform arithmetic on large numbers. In addition, the larger the word size—assuming that the bus can transmit a single word in a single cycle—the less time it takes to move data from the memory to the CPU where it is processed. Word processing applications gain little from the arithmetic advantage of a 16-bit computer versus an 8-bit machine, but they may gain from the increased data transmission rates afforded by a 16-bit bus.

There is another advantage of a larger word-size machine. The amount of computer memory that can be directly accessed in a single cycle depends upon the word size. It is usually advantageous to be able to access as large a span of memory as possible. Even for word processing applications, it helps if you can keep most of the pages you are working on in the computer random access memory rather than on disk.

The amount of memory you can access in a single cycle depends upon the size of the address register in the CPU. If the address register is 16 bits, you can access only 64,000 bytes in a single cycle. Consequently, many computers have a maximum memory size of 64K. With a 24-bit address register, we can access a million bytes; with 32 bits, 4 billion bytes.

The larger word-size machines also have an advantage in executing programs. Presume that an 8-bit computer is going to execute the machine instructions shown above. In this case, each CPU processing cycle can only read, write, or alter 8 bits at a time. Assume that A, B, C are integers stored as 16 binary bits (two bytes). The computer would take 16 steps [as shown in Table 1a] to execute the program's three instructions. Each step requires at least one computer cycle. If you were using a 16-bit computer, each address, plus the numbers A, B, and C, would be in a single word. In Table 1b, you can see that the ability to read and write 16-bit words reduces the number of steps to nine.

Now it should be clear that if the number of processing cycles per second is constant, then a 16-bit computer will be faster than its 8-bit counterpart. Why? It processes both instructions and data by accessing fewer words, and each access numbers one processing cycle. Fewer processing cycles means more speed. If all processing were character-oriented, the improvement would not be as dramatic, because the size of the logical units (bytes) is the same as the size of the physical units (8-bit words). However, if your applications involve many computations with floating point numbers, then a 32-bit processor will be far superior.

SOME FINAL WORDS

We have taken liberties to simplify this tutorial. We suggested, e.g., that two bytes are needed to identify a particular word in a 64K memory space. Yet, if we deal with blocks of memory in which all words have the same 8 high-order (or leftmost) bits, then we simply identify a unique address by providing the low-order (or rightmost) 8 bits. This is called "paging with a 256-word page." All words are accessed in relation to the start of a known page number.

Once the paging scheme is used, the pages need not be stored in sequential order but may be treated independently. With "virtual memory" each page is in fact treated independently. When the program requires instructions or data from a page, that page is loaded into memory. If no space is available, then the new page is written over another page which the system software "guesses" will no longer be used. In this way, you can run programs too large to fit completely into memory at one time. Hence the term "virtual."

Just as paging is used to identify words in a 64K memory using only 8 bits, a special register, called a "segment register," is used in some machines to address words in memories larger than 64K. The true address is computed by adding the contents of this register to the 16-bit address. As we have seen, addresses in memory are designated with very large binary numbers whose bits are grouped in sets of four. Each set represents 16 possible combinations which can be written 0,1,2,3,. . .9,A,B,C,D,E,F with 0 for all zero bits and F for all one bits. Thus, we have a "hexadecimal" number system with a base of 16. Hexadecimal digits, of course, can be added and subtracted and they provide another convenient notation system for representing binary numbers. For example, a 16-bit address may be represented as four hexadecimal digits.

Finally, you should note that a 32-bit floating point number does not have enough accuracy for some computations. For example, in summing the squares of a very large or very small number, you may find that your result has only three or four digits of accuracy. If this is insufficient, a 64-bit number (8 bytes) can be used. To maintain accuracy, 7 of the bytes make up the mantissa. This is called "double precision floating point format." Some computers even support triple precision.

We have alluded to the word size as being a single attribute of the computer. If the computer has a 16-bit bus and 16-bit general-purpose registers, all would agree it is a 16-bit computer. But what if the computer had 16-bit general-purpose registers, a 24-bit address register and an 8-bit bus, as is the case with the Intel 8088 used in the IBM PC? This is usually referred to as a 16-bit computer although it can only fetch one character at a time from memory; yet it can address a total of one million bytes of memory. This machine would be more accurately described as a 16/8-bit machine. The Motorola 68000 is sometimes described as a 32-bit machine because many of its registers are 32 bits long; however, it has only a 16-bit bus. The lesson here is not to accept a simple definition of a computer's word size. Ask about the bus size, the register size, and the addressing scheme to get a good understanding of the computer potential.

PROGRAMMING LANGUAGES

BRUCE I. BLUM

Computer technology has two physical aspects: the *hardware* which tirelessly and rapidly repeats simple operations, and the *software* which sequences those operations to produce a useful tool. The software, in turn, can be divided into two categories. The *systems software* is that collection of programs which allows the user to interact with and create programs for the hardware. It is usually purchased with the hardware. The other class of software, *applications*, consists of programs which perform special functions such as word processing, accounting, or billing for the user.

A *program* is defined as a set of complete instructions which tells the computer how to perform some function for a user. Creating a program is called *programming* or *coding* (writing code). Think of writing a program as using a special language to explain something to the computer. In fact, this special language is a true language with syntax and semantics. However, unlike human languages which grow and develop more or less capriciously, computer languages are usually planned and developed consciously to meet specific needs and solve particular programming problems.

SOME BACKGROUND ON PROGRAMMING LANGUAGES

Hardware is limited in what it can do, which means that program-

BRUCE I. BLUM

Bruce I. Blum has over 20 years experience in developing information systems. He's a member of the Principal Professional Staff of the Johns Hopkins Applied Physics Laboratory and also an Associate Professor of Biomedical Engineering at the School of Medicine.

From 1975 to 1983, Mr. Blum was the director of the Clinical Information Systems Division of the Department of Biomedical Engineering. He was responsible for the design and implementation of major clinical information systems for the Oncology Center and for the Outpatient Department.

Mr. Blum was the Program Chair for the Sixth Annual Symposium on Computer Applications in Medical Care (SCAMC-82), and is the editor of the new Springer-Verlag series Readings in Computers in Medicine. *He received a B.S. from Rutgers University in 1951, an M.A. in History from Columbia University in 1954, and an M.A. in Mathematics from the University of Maryland in 1965. He teaches computer science at the Johns Hopkins School of Engineering.*

ming languages must be very explicit and concise. Each programming language has its advantages and disadvantages. Some are more efficient for the computer to execute, while others are easier for the user to learn, and still others may be clumsy to program but easy to read, especially for a non-programmer.

The maxim is often true: when you've met the parent you can better understand the child. This tutorial will introduce you to three computer languages that are in some sense parents to all modern languages. Simple examples using the coding style of each language will give you a sense of how they look and flow.

The First Languages

Back in the days of the very first computers, storage was limited. Each computer program was a sequence of process control steps; these were coded in terms the computer could readily process—binary sequences of ones and zeroes—and recorded on paper tape in terms of the presence and absence of holes. This was a laborious and error-prone approach. Computer memory was treated as a long string of locations, each assigned a unique number. Programmers accessing a location had to punch in the location number they desired.

As computers began to grow in size and power, programs were written to translate the programmer's wishes into computer commands. For example, if the binary sequence 010110 were interpreted by the computer as an instruction to add the contents of two registers, the programmer could enter the mnemonic phrase "ADD" and the program would substitute this binary sequence. The program that did this was called an assembler, and assembly language became the first true programming language.

Assembly Languages

Instructions written in assembly languages are very similar to those which are internally available to a computer's central processor (CPU). In fact, assembly languages are not standard; they vary with the hardware for which they were designed. To illustrate a typical assembly language, let us assume that we have an extremely simple computer. Suppose we wish to add two numbers and store the result as a third number. The computer would have to execute the following sequence of steps:

- Bring the value for A to a register (a special storage location of the computer where computations may be performed).
- Add the value for B to the contents of the register. (This puts the sum into the register, supplanting the value of A.)
- Store the resulting sum C into a memory location.

We might write this in assembly language program (using a register called R1) as:

```
LOAD  R1,A
ADD   R1,B
STORE R1,C
```

Notice that in the above example we have used the letters A, B, and C as symbols (variable names) which stand for the values contained in certain memory locations. This is reminiscent of high school algebra problems: "Let X equal. . . ," where X symbolizes a value. The values are stored as binary sequences in one or more "words" of the computer's memory. (A word is the most convenient number of bits for a particular computer to deal with. The Apple IIe uses 8-bit words, the IBM-PC uses 16-bit words, the Apple Macintosh and Lisa use 16- or 32-bit words. A unit of 8 bits is called a byte.)

A major feature of assembly language is that it allows us to think of storage as a set of variables and not solely as a sequence of words of computer memory. Assembly language permits us to assign names to memory locations.

FORTRAN PROVIDES THE SUBROUTINE TO ALLOW THE PROGRAMMER TO WRITE A SMALL PROGRAM ONCE AND USE IT IN MANY PLACES WITHIN A LARGER PROGRAM, CALLED SDEV.

A PROGRAMMING MODEL

Virtually all programming languages are simply different ways to translate a sequence of user-defined steps into a sequence of actions performed by the computer on its memory contents. For example, the BASIC statement:

```
Let C = A + B
```

accomplishes the same task as the previous assembly language program.

In order to understand any programming language, whether FORTRAN, BASIC, or some other, it is best to have a conceptual model of how the computer works. The programming language then becomes a user-oriented expression of activities within that model. We can think of a computer system as containing four major components:

- *The Central Processing Unit (CPU).* This performs the actual computations. The language statements describe what the CPU is to do.
- *Working Storage or Memory.* This holds the programs and data currently being used. All variables (e.g., A, B, C) are retained here. On most microcomputers, working storage is lost when the power is shut off.
- *Secondary Storage.* This is also called permanent storage. It permits information to be maintained in machine-readable form over a long duration. Common secondary storage media are floppy disks, cassette tapes, magnetic tapes, and hard disks. The CPU transfers data to and from permanent storage by performing input/output (I/O) operations.

■ *User Communication.* This is a special type of input/output oriented towards the user. Examples are keyboard input, mouse, or touch-screen input, and screen, printer output, or voice output.

The CPU

The assembly-language program and BASIC program given above are functionally the same. In BASIC, a high-order language (HOL), the user specified what was to be done and the internal processes of the language took care of assigning memory locations. In assembly, a low-order language (LOL), the user had to specify which register the CPU should use. There are many different high-order languages. The major differences among them are based upon their view of the kinds of problems their users wish to solve.

Working Storage

Working storage contains both the program being run and the data used by the program. One of the key requirements for a programming language is that it should manage the data in working storage. The user references data by name, and the programming language maps that name into storage locations.

You can think of variable names as labels for "bins." The bin may consist of one, two, or more computer words, but as a programmer you do not need to be concerned with how the programming language assigns words to bins. The statement

```
C = A + B
```

can now be expressed as: get the contents from the bin labeled A, add it to the contents of the bin labeled B, and store the result in the bin labeled C. Bins A and B are unchanged. You need not be concerned with the actual physical location of the bins.

Secondary Storage

Secondary storage is much larger than working storage. It is used to save programs and data. Because it is so large, it is organized physically into "blocks" consisting of hundreds of words. The precise size of a block depends on the storage device. A floppy disk, for example, uses 128- or 256-byte blocks, while a giant UNIVAC mainframe uses a 10,000-byte block. Here again, in programming you need not be concerned with the physical blocks; instead, you deal with "records" which are part of a "file." For example, you might define a *file* containing separate records for each patient, with each *record* containing a single patient's name, sex, and birth date. A record might be smaller or larger than the storage device's block, but you do not have to worry about this. The programming language takes care of assigning the appropriate number of blocks or partial blocks to each record.

Files are managed by the operating system which, in most cases, is independent of the programming language. However every programming language must have the ability to read records from and write records into files. In many languages, the same read and write statements used for file records are also used for other I/O operations.

COBOL'S STRENGTH IS ITS ABILITY TO DEFINE THE DATA STRUCTURES HELD IN SECONDARY STORAGE—THE ONLY PLACE WITH ROOM FOR THE MASSIVE DATA REQUIRED FOR BUSINESS APPLICATIONS.

User Communication

High-level languages have commands to permit input and output of data. BASIC uses INPUT, LINE INPUT, WRITE, and PRINT. The transfer of data from the machine to a form usable by the human operator is called writing or output; transferring data from the user to a machine-usable form is called reading or input. I will discuss the writing process; reading is analogous.

To write data, the machine must convert data from the internal binary representation to printable characters. The programming language provides the capability to position the characters on the page or screen. Most languages also permit detailed specifications of the format of the output:

```
PRINT "The end"
PRINT using "###.#",X
```

These are both examples in BASIC. The first statement prints the string "The end". The second is an example of a format statement. The string "###.#" tells the computer to print the number contained in the variable X, using 3 digits to the left of the decimal point and rounding to one place on the right of the decimal. Many languages also let you indicate exactly where information is to be printed on the output page (or screen). For a statement which is read, the format indicates how the input is to be coded into binary sequences and assigned to variables, e.g., whether it is to be regarded as text or a number, whether the data is read left-justified or right-justified, whether there is an assumed decimal place, and so on.

SOME MAINFRAME PROGRAMMING LANGUAGES

The languages used in today's microcomputers are derived from those used in the large computers of the 1960s. There are three main languages of interest: FORTRAN, COBOL, and ALGOL. FORTRAN had a profound impact on the design of BASIC. Because of their continuing usefulness, FORTRAN and COBOL are now available on many microcomputer systems. COBOL is the most heavily used language for mainframe computers. ALGOL, though not widely available on microcomputers, was a major influence on some newer languages, such as PASCAL and C, which are widely available on microcomputers. Each of these three languages has a distinctive style and qualities which make it better for some uses than the other languages.

FORTRAN Concepts

The FORmula TRANslating System, or FORTRAN, was first specified in 1954 as an alternative to assembly languages. After five years of development and several versions of the language, FORTRAN was implemented and became widely accepted. It is the most commonly used language for scientific programming ("number crunching"). It is a highly standardized language; consequently, transfer of ANSII standard FORTRAN between machines of different vendors is easy. Furthermore, it introduced several concepts which are central to understanding programming languages.

DATA TYPES

One of the functions of a programming language is to manage different types of data—for example, text strings and numbers—in working storage. There are several ways of representing numbers in working storage, and each method creates a different type of data. Some data types require more than one word; some CPU instructions can be applied to certain data types and not to others. One of FORTRAN's contributions was to provide programmers with a convenient method for allocating working storage to different types of data.

Some common data types are:

- Integer: This is a positive or negative whole number, usually less than 32,768.
- Floating Point: This is a real number written in the form of scientific notation. It generally varies in size from 10^{-38} to 10^{+38}.
- Double Precision: This is a real number, similar in format to the floating point number except that double precision uses more bits and thus can store data more accurately. Some implementations permit even larger numbers than 10^{+38} to be stored.
- Character: Later versions of FORTRAN added this data type to permit convenient definition of strings of characters.

FORTRAN initially assumed that

A *FORTRAN* SUBROUTINE

Figure 1. A sample subroutine for computing the standard deviation of N values.

```
      SUBROUTINE STDEV(V,N,STD)
C
C     V is an array with N numbers previously defined in
C        the main program
C     STD is computed by this routine
C
      DIMENSION V(30)
C
C     The next 4 lines of code compute the mean
      SUM=0
      DO 10 I=1,N
      SUM=SUM + V(I)
   10 CONTINUE
      MEAN=SUM/N
C
C     Now the standard deviation is computed by summing
C        the square of differences from the mean
C
      NMINUS=N-1
      VSUM=0
      DO 20 I=1,N
      VSUM=VSUM + (V(I)-MEAN)**2
   20 CONTINUE
      VAR=VSUM/NMINUS
C
C     The standard deviation is the square root of the variance;
C     SQRT is a FORTRAN library function which computes
C        square roots
C
      STD=SQRT(VAR)
      RETURN
```

NOTES ON THE *FORTRAN* EXAMPLE

- The SUBROUTINE statement declares that this is a part of a program rather than a complete freestanding package. Some pieces of information ("parameters") are supplied by the main program. These parameters are called V, N, and STD within the subroutine. N will be the number of values, V will be an array which contains the values, and STD will be the standard deviation which is computed by the subroutine.
- Lines in FORTRAN with a "C" in column one are comments. These should be used liberally to make the code readable.
- The DIMENSION V(30) specifies that V is an array which uses only one subscript. Statements which reference V(I) are accessing the value which is in the "Ith" location of V.
- The "DO 10 I=1,N" statement is used to loop. It will cause all lines of code up to and including statement number 10 to be executed N times. First I will equal 1; then I is set to 2, then 3, etc.
- The RETURN statement marks the end of the subroutine. Control returns to the place in the program that accessed the subroutine.

any variable name that started with I, J, K, L, M, or N was an integer; anything else was a floating point. Thus the computer would automatically assume that a variable called "NUMBER" would be an integer (no decimal place), and a variable called "RATIO" would be regarded as a floating point number because its first letter is not one of those listed above. Later commands were added to allow the programmer to identify a variable as belonging to a specific data type, regardless of its name, including double precision, complex numbers, alphabetics, etc.

ARRAYS

The first computers were developed for military ballistics calculation, so the first programming languages were oriented toward computation. Because most calculations required frequent reference to large tables of numbers, FORTRAN provides a technique for users to do this easily. That concept—being able to refer to tables of data using symbolic names—is one of FORTRAN's most significant contributions. The same fundamental method was borrowed by BASIC, PASCAL, ALGOL, and C.

In FORTRAN (and most other programming languages) we refer to a table as an array. Before using an array, you have to tell the computer how big it is to be, so that the program can allocate it the correct number of storage bins. You do this with a dimension statement.

```
DIMENSION VECTOR(7), MATRIX(3,7),
ARRAY(3,7,3)
```

This defines three arrays: a one-dimensional array (VECTOR), a 3×7 array called MATRIX, and a three-dimensional array called ARRAY. Later in the program we can reference specific elements within these arrays with statements such as:

```
A = VECTOR(3) + MATRIX(1,2)
B = ARRAY(I,J,K)
```

In these statements, A is set to the sum of the third element of VECTOR and the first-column second-row element of MATRIX. B is set to the value in ARRAY located by I, J, and K (variables defined elsewhere in the program).

IT WAS NEVER REALLY USED MUCH, BUT ALGOL IS IMPORTANT BECAUSE IT SO STRONGLY INFLUENCED MODERN PROGRAMMING LANGUAGES INCLUDING C AND PASCAL.

COMPUTATIONS

In assembly language, programmers were required to reference variables in the order in which the machine had to process them. Frequently, this was not the "natural" way that people think of a problem. FORTRAN permitted programmers to define computations as formulas the way scientists and engineers had always done. For example:

```
A = (B + C + D) * 56/E - 23
```

The only thing unusual about this equation is that the multiply operation is signified by an asterisk (*), not a times sign (×). The above statement instructs the computer first to add variables B, C, and D together. The result is multiplied by 56, then divided by variable E. Finally, 23 is subtracted, and the result stored into variable A. Parentheses are used to specify the order of computation. This type of computational definition is now part of virtually all computer languages.

FLOW CONTROL

Each statement in FORTRAN can be labeled with a number. (Note that BASIC modified this rule so that *every* statement *had* to be given a number.) To branch or jump from one statement to another, one uses the GOTO command (just as in BASIC). For example:

```
GOTO 100
```

This tells the computer to skip to the statement labeled "100". Most languages provide some analogous statement for jumping to a specific line of code. However, GOTO statements result in "spaghetti code" that is difficult to follow. Most computer scientists try to avoid the GOTO statement. (They use nested branching statements or subroutines, discussed below.)

To repeat a sequence of steps one or more times, you use a loop or iteration. All computer languages provide some tools for accomplishing this extremely common computer task. For processing a loop, FORTRAN provides the DO statement illustrated below.

```
Compute the sum of 10,11,12,...20 with
          NSUM = 0
          DO 1 I = 10, 20
    1     NSUM = NSUM + I
```

The line labeled 1 will be executed 11 times: first with I set to 10, then set to 11, and on until I equals 20. The sum will be placed into variable NSUM. The DO statement provides a compact way of repeating a series of statements.

OTHER FLOW CONTROL STATEMENTS

Another common control structure is the conditional branch. It is an IF/THEN statement:

```
IF some condition is true THEN do this; ELSE do
that.
```

In FORTRAN, the IF statement has undergone changes with various versions of the language. The earliest versions allowed the programmer only to GOTO (branch) to statements if an expression was less than, equal to, or greater than zero. For example:

```
IF (X - 3/Y) 10, 20, 30
```

This statement tells the computer to evaluate X − 3/Y. If the value is less than zero it will jump to statement 10; if equal to zero, it will jump to statement 20; and if greater than zero, it will jump to statement 30. The above DO loop could also be written with an IF statement as follows.

```
    NSUM = 0
    I = 10
1   NSUM =
    NSUM + I
    I = I + 1
    If(I - 20) 1,
    1, 2
2   -----------
    ---         (Next line of code in program)
```

However, I would not encourage this practice because the DO loop is a simpler and easier-to-read construct for iteration.

SUBROUTINES

The computation of a standard deviation is not particularly difficult. If we have to do it often, however, we might wish to write it once and then reference that program each time we need to compute a standard deviation. FORTRAN provides the subroutine to allow the programmer to write a small program once and use it in many places within a larger program, called SDEV. An example is the subroutine for computing the standard deviation of N values (see Figure 1).

A collection of subroutines is called a library. The ability to build and share program libraries adds to the power of a system. Because FORTRAN developed as a natural way for scientists and engineers to write mathematical expressions, they soon built large libraries of mathematical subroutines which they could link together in order to produce the programs that solved their problems. Most implementations come with a large collection of mathematical functions (trigonometric, exponential, etc.). In addition, commercial libraries are available for statistical analysis, graphics, and other uses. This enormous investment in program libraries and training has made FORTRAN a popular programming language even to this day.

AN *ALGOL* PROGRAM

Figure 2. An ALGOL program to compute a standard deviation.

```
procedure STDV(V,N);value N;
   real array V;integer N;
   begin integer I,NMO;real SSUM,AVER,VAR
   SSUM: = 0;
   for i: = 1 step 1 until N do SSUM: = SSUM + V[I];
   AVER: = SSUM/N;
   NMO: = N - 1;
   SSUM: = 0;
   for i: = 1 step 1 until N do SSUM: = SSUM + (V[I] - AVER) ^ 2;
   VAR: = SSUM/NMO;
   STDV: = VAR ^ .5;
end;
```

NOTES ON THE *ALGOL* PROGRAM

- This is a procedure which assumes that N has already been set to a count of items and V[I] has been set to their value. Note that ALGOL and FORTRAN permit "argument passing," while BASIC does not.
- The specification of V as an array alerts the ALGOL compiler that storage will be needed. The actual allocation is done in the routine that creates the data.
- The syntax for looping ("for i:=1 step 1 until N") is analogous to the BASIC FOR and FORTRAN DO loops.
- ALGOL uses the operator "=" for TESTING whether two values are equal. It uses ":=" for ASSIGNING one variable to equal an expression.

COBOL: A Different View

FORTRAN worked well for computation, but it was not effective for business applications. FORTRAN was designed to do a lot of processing on a modest number of records (that which would fit in working storage). Commercial applications, on the other hand, needed to do a little bit of processing on each of a large number of records. A different language was required. The COmmon Business Oriented Language (COBOL) was implemented in 1960 as a standard language which could be used by all the military branches. It was designed to be self-documenting and highly transportable. Each program is divided into four divisions:

- IDENTIFICATION DIVISION: A description of the program.
- ENVIRONMENT DIVISION: A description of the hardware and file names used.
- DATA DIVISION: A description of the data structures to be processed.
- PROCEDURE DIVISION: The processing logic.

Because the language was intended to be used by business analysts, the syntax favors explicitness over scientific conciseness. The following statements might appear in a PROCEDURE DIVISION:

```
SUBTRACT 7 FROM X GIVING Y
DIVIDE 13 INTO X GIVING Q REMAINDER R
DIVIDE X INTO Y ROUNDED
```

DATA STRUCTURES

Brevity is not COBOL's strong suit. Compared to the formulas FORTRAN uses for algebraic computations, the example above is clumsy and wordy. COBOL's strength is its ability to define the data structures held in secondary storage—the only place with room for the large amounts of data required for business applications. (The original version of FORTRAN had no such capability. More recent versions of FORTRAN do, but not with the power and flexibility of COBOL's approach.)

Now look at how COBOL performs a common business job—putting out a bill. Each bill would include two major components: the printed heading which identifies the customer, date, and salesman; and the detail which identifies the name, quantity, and costs for each item entered.

A definition of this structure in the DATA DIVISION might be:

```
01 BILL.
  02 HEADING.
    03 CUSTOMER-NUMBER PICTURE 9999.
    03 DATE.
      04 MONTH PICTURE 99.
      04 DAY PICTURE 99.
      04 YEAR PICTURE 99.
    03 SALESMAN-NUMBER PICTURE 9999.
    03 ITEM-COUNT PICTURE 99.
  02 ITEMS OCCURS 1 TO 99 TIMES
       DEPENDING ON ITEM-COUNT.
    03 ITEM-NAME PICTURE X(40).
    03 ITEM-QUANT PICTURE 999.
    03 ITEM-COST PICTURE 9999V99.
```

The programmer assigns a number (01, 02, 03, 04. . .) to indicate the hierarchical relationship among elements in the data structures. The PICTURE phrase indicates the data type, and is used to validate the data. For example, the numeral 9 indicates numeric data. X(40) in ITEM-NAME indicates a 40-character string of alphanumerics. The V in the ITEM-COST definition indicates a decimal point, so its value can range up to $9999.99. As you can see from these examples, with a little explanation, the program is easy to understand.

Surveys show that almost half of all programs are written in COBOL. The reasons for its resiliency are connected with its position of precedence in history: a vast library of COBOL applications already exists, and a large number of skilled COBOL programmers has been trained.

A *BASIC* PROGRAM FOR STANDARD DEVIATION

```
2000    REM Compute Mean & Standard Deviation
2010    REM Must have N= number of items
2020    REM          X(1), X(2), X(3), . . X(N) = values
2030    REM          defined previously.
2040    REM First compute Mean
2050  SUM=0
2060  FOR I=1 TO N
2070    SUM=SUM+X(I)
2080    NEXT I
2090  MEAN=SUM/N
2100    REM     Now compute Standard Deviation
2110  NMINUS1=N-1
2120  SUM=0
2130  FOR I=1 TO N
2140    SUM=SUM + (X(I)-MEAN)^2
2150    NEXT I
2160  VAR=SUM/NMINUS1        This is the variance
2170  STD=SQR(VAR)
2180  PRINT "The mean is ";MEAN;" and standard deviation is";
2190  PRINT USING "###.####";STD
2200  RETURN
```

POINTS OF INTEREST IN THE *BASIC* PROGRAM

- **Lines 2050–2090 compute the mean (average).**
- **Line 2060 initiates a loop using variable I; line 2080 denotes the end of lines within the loop.**
- **Lines 2110–2170 compute the standard deviation.**
- **In line 2140, the mean is subtracted from each number, the remainder is squared (the "^2" operator), and a running total is kept.**
- **Line 2160 computes the variance. The standard deviation is the square root of the variance.**
- **General note: Multiple commands could have been placed onto single lines but were not, for reasons of clarity. Likewise, there are more efficient methods for computation that were not used for the same reason.**

An Overview of ALGOL

The final mainframe programming language of historical interest is ALGOL. It was never really used much, but is important because it so strongly influenced modern programming languages including C and PASCAL. The creation of an ALGOrithmic Language (ALGOL) was begun in the late 1950s by an international committee of computer scientists. A version was published in 1960—ALGOL60—which was not widely used. It *was* frequently used by computer scientists in their published work, however. It was the language in which examples of a new, more efficient computer technique were written.

ALGOL60 was designed to facilitate the expression of logical flow by expanding upon the control structures provided by FORTRAN. Programs were written in free text form, using indentation to suggest program structure. Processing units are written as blocks (different from the block used by the computer program to write information to storage) which start with a command (BEGIN, DO) and terminate with an "END". The use of this block structuring permits the physical layout of a program listing to reflect to some degree the actual logical flow of the program. The iteration (DO) statement is much more general, and allows the loop to continue while a condition is true. For an example of an ALGOL program, see Figure 2, a program to compute a standard deviation.

ALGOL provided a common language for computer scientists, and influenced the way they thought about programming. This ALGOL style has become an integral part of the block-structured languages, for example PL/1, PASCAL, C, and ADA.

SUMMARY

This tutorial has very simply examined the general structure of computers and programming languages, and briefly described the three major historical programming languages: FORTRAN, COBOL, and ALGOL. From the outset, the goals of these three languages were different. FORTRAN was designed to facilitate computation and to be easy for scientists and engineers to use. These are the same features which eventually made BASIC so popular in our microcomputers. COBOL was designed to manage large files; while it is available for some microcomputers, it has little applicability to the small-computer environment. Finally, ALGOL was designed to implement the building blocks of programming systems—the algorithms. The style it created is easily recognized in PASCAL.

After some 25 years of programming-language history, the features of the languages have tended to merge together. Still, there are clear distinctions. Two common programming languages—BASIC and PASCAL—were first developed as students' learning tools. Each has grown in power; each also provides a different view of program constructions. As microcomputers have become more powerful, other languages have become available. There are many programming languages to choose from, and no one is the "best." I hope this tutorial has provided some insight to help you in selecting the languages best suited to your applications. □

COMPUTER-AIDED EDUCATION

RAY E. EBERTS, Ph.D.

When television first came out thirty years ago, educators thought it would transform teaching. Since it could present material cheaply to a wide audience, students would not have to travel far for education. Today, television is still used in teaching, but it has never quite reached its vast potential. Perhaps one reason television teaching has not been more effective is that students cannot interact with it as they would with a teacher.

Interactive computers are now perceived much the way television was thirty years ago; they can present instruction cheaply to students at remote sites. In addition, the computer is interactive, eliminating one of television's main problems. It can also perform some tasks quicker and better than a teacher. One researcher [1] compares the potential educational impact of interactive computers to that of printing. Books could reproduce the instructional material. Computers can do that, and also reproduce the instructional interactions (feedback, scoring, branching, and record keeping). In theory, therefore, the best instructors' techniques can be replicated.

RAY E. EBERTS, Ph.D.
Ray Eberts is an assistant professor in the School of Industrial Engineering at Purdue University, with a Ph.D. in cognitive psychology from the University of Illinois. Before going to Purdue, he worked at Honeywell in Minneapolis, where he was involved in the design and construction of computer-aided instruction.

Educators already use computers heavily. A November 1984 estimate showed 600,000 computers in elementary and secondary schools. This is one computer for every 66 students—a twentyfold increase since 1980.

PLATO (Programmed Logic for Automated Teaching Operations) is one of the largest educational computer systems. It was developed at the University of Illinois, and is marketed by Control Data Corporation. Over $900 million has been invested in its research and development. It is heavily used. Between July 1974 and September 1981, students and instructors clocked roughly 9,600,000 hours of use. There are over 12,000 instructional hours available in more than 150 subject areas. At the University of Delaware, 9,000 students take 112 courses each semester on the PLATO system.

PLATO has been used to teach basic sciences as well as medical school coursework. The University of Illinois and the University of Ohio have invested heavily in computer-aided education for medical students. Recently, Harvard University inaugurated what they call "New Pathways," an approach to medical education that uses computers heavily. Massachusetts General Hospital and the University of Seattle have developed extensive computer-based aids for postgraduate education. (For further information on these systems, contact the addresses at the end of this article.)

Despite these successes, many questions remain. What kinds of instructional materials are ideal for computer-aided education? How much time is required to program the instruction? How effective will it be compared to traditional methods? If you are the learner, would you prefer the computer or the manual approach? If you are the teacher, will the effort of creating a computer-aided course be worthwhile?

CHARACTERISTICS OF COMPUTER-AIDED EDUCATION

Computer-aided education comes in many forms, which vary with the degree of computer involvement in the instructional process. In *computer-managed instruction*, the computer's role is primarily administrative; it registers students, upgrades test forms, and maintains student grade files. In *computer-assisted instruction* (CAI) and *computer-based instruction* (CBI), the computer performs some of the instructional tasks while the human teacher provides others. *Intelligent computer-assisted instruction* takes over an even larger share of the instructor's tasks, including tutoring, natural-lan-

COURSEWARE FOR THE IBM-PC*

Table 1

Software	Vendor	Features	Price
The Author (64K)	Raptor Systems, Inc. Stillwater, MN	Graphics Monochrome Record keeping Function keys	$295
CAI*Plus (256K)	EduCaitor, Inc. Groton, CT	Not available	$500
Easylearn (128K)	Miracle Computing Lawrence, KS	Create text materials Color or monochrome Preprogrammed word 32,000 screens	$250
HyperGraphics	HyperGraphics Corporation Richardson, TX	Color graphics board Monitor	$395
IAS (128K)	McGraw-Hill New York, NY	Color Video (VCR) Menu-based	$1,500
Med-Caps	Health Sciences Consortium Carrboro, NC	Not available	Not available
Micropac (64K)	Microsystems Software Ltd. Tempe, AZ	Two drives Printer	Available free with selected texts from Wadsworth Publishing

*This information is adapted from [2] and [3].

guage question-answering, and guidance, so that computers can be administrators, assistants, or full-fledged "teachers."

Instructional material provided by the computer is called *courseware*, and it is generally produced with the help of special programs called *authoring systems*. When a teacher or programmer has used these to produce some courseware, it can later be edited or revised by the same authoring programs. The authoring programs take care of administrative details of instruction, such as branching and record keeping, and free the author from having to deal with the morass of programming details that would be needed if BASIC or PASCAL were used to write the lesson. Commercial authoring packages are available for both large and small computers. (See Table 1 for a sample of authoring coursework currently available for the IBM-PC.)

An important part of the courseware is computer feedback in response to student inputs. This feedback can range from a simple "right" or "wrong" to a complex analysis indicating "how right" or "how wrong." And the feedback computerized instruction provides is extremely effective because of its immediacy. Some experimental techniques even analyze the student's problem-solving strategies and critique them for his or her benefit.

The courseware can also adapt itself to the level of an individual student. In adaptive instruction, task characteristics are automatically changed from simple to complex depending on the student's facility with the task. This is important, because if the instruction is too difficult, students may give up; if it is too easy, they may become bored. Whether the student or the program should control the sequence of instruction is an important research issue. Experimental evidence suggests that students have trouble choosing the correct level of instructional difficulty; consequently, this task should probably be managed by the computer—which can adjust the amount of instruction, the sequence, and the instructional display time, all according to feedback from the student.

The actual system used by a student consists of both software and hardware. *Delivery-system software* presents the material developed by the authoring system, and controls the student/computer interaction. Specifically, the delivery system uses the courseware to provide information to the student, asks questions about it, and

Software	Vendor	Features	Price
Microtim	JL Educational and Computer Services, Inc. Dallas, TX	Not available	$1,400
PC-CME (128K)	Computers in Patient Care Little Rock, AR	For use with one drive	$10
PC/PILOT (64K)	Washington Computer Services Bellingham, WA	Color or monochrome Graphics editor	$100
Private Tutor (Version 2.00)	Centers selling IBM products	Not available	$50
Teacher's Quiz Designer	Centers selling IBM products	Not available	$75
Teacher Turned Author! (128K)	Raster Technology Longwood, FL	Menu-driven Color of monochrome Color graphics Record keeping	$399–999
TenCORE (128K)	Computer Teaching Corporation Champaign, IL	Color Graphics	$2,000
Test Management System (128K)	Wilson T. Price & Stephen Brown	Two drives Printer	Available free with selected texts from Holt, Rinehart & Winston
Total Recall	Custom Data Services, Cromwell, CT	Not available	$79.95

then moves to succeeding stages of the lesson, depending upon the student's understanding at each step. Delivery system hardware can include off-line adjunctive materials like images or sounds on computer-controlled devices, such as audio tape or disk, videotape, and microfiche. In other cases, the material simply references workbooks or handbooks available to the student.

COMPUTERIZED EDUCATION VERSUS LIVE EDUCATION

The relative evaluation of educational methods is inherently difficult due to problems with outcome measures and with obtaining adequate controls. Anyone trying to compare computerized courses to manual courses should consider these problems, as well as differences in the quality of the course material taught by humans and computers.

Studies that have compared the two have demonstrated the whole range of results: sometimes the computer-taught are better; sometimes the human teaching is better, and sometimes neither approach shows an advantage. Again, the conclusion depends somewhat on the material being taught. Computers are better at drill and practice, simulations, and interactive graphics. Teachers are better at tutoring and responding to questions [4].

Although teaching effectiveness is difficult to measure, computers show clear advantages in the relatively easy-to-measure area of instructional cost. The University of Delaware performed the most extensive estimate of the cost of computer systems, focusing on PLATO [5]. In 1982, the cost per terminal hour for a student was $2.47 for a large mainframe PLATO system, and $1.15 for smaller versions using microcomputers (MICRO PLATO). It is difficult to estimate the comparable cost for live instruction because this depends on the class size and the material being presented, but one estimate for a college instructor in 1984 was $3 to $7 per student contact hour [5]. Computers save time for the student by individualizing instruction. Several comparative studies show that computer-taught students could cover the given material 14–66% faster (see Table 2). These data suggest that in a classroom, the slowest learners tend to limit the speed at which material can be covered; but in a computerized system, the individual student can move at his own pace. This savings in student time has special cost advantages when students are being paid for their

REDUCTION IN INSTRUCTION TIME DUE TO INDIVIDUALIZATION*

Table 2

Percent Reduction in Time to Complete	Description
66	Training at United Airlines [7]
64	Average from evaluation of military systems [8]
63	Technical maintenance training at American Airlines [7]
50–67	Computerized courses in school districts [9]
40	College courses [10]
33	Course at Federal Aviation Administration [11]
15–27	Navy advanced maintenance course [12]
15–25	Navy apprentice training [12]

* This information is taken from [6].

learning time, as in on-the-job training.

Computer-aided education systems have obvious advantages for record keeping. The computer does the grading, assigns instructional modules, and records attendance, freeing the instructor's time for more student contact.

DESIGN AND EVALUATION OF COMPUTERIZED EDUCATION

Many educators are placed in the position of having to design or evaluate courseware for computer-aided education. These processes must be based on a consideration of the kinds of learning strategies a medical student uses to master a certain subject.

Students do employ a wide variety of strategies to master an assigned task or subject, and good teachers generally guide the student to the appropriate learning strategy for the material at hand. For example, learning to make a diagnosis requires a problem-solving strategy; learning straight facts requires a drill-and-practice strategy. Computer-aided education is better for some learning strategies than others. Before embarking on the development of a computer-aided course, be sure that the best learning strategy for the material involved can be implemented by the available course-authoring system. Table 3 provides a summary of major learning strategies, and rates their ease of application through available authoring systems.

"Drill and practice" is a simple, obvious learning strategy which is important to medical subject matter. Proficiency in most medical fields requires considerable practice, much of which comes with experience in the field; for example, the expertise of a senior radiologist comes from experience in reading as many as half a million radiographs. Computers are excellent at providing the practice needed to become proficient in many medical subjects.

Motivation is also important in the learning process. Computers can apply a variety of motivation techniques, including video-game-type graphics, competition, automatic adaptation of difficulty levels, and multilevel goals. Many courseware authoring systems come with a graphics capability. The introduction of other techniques (such as competition) often requires special programming.

Learning by example is an especially effective teaching method. The instructor provides a specific example, and then derives a general rule from it. This teaching strategy is easy to implement through existing courseware-authoring systems.

Learning by analogy is similar to learning by example. The instructor chooses a concrete situation familiar to the student and presents new information in related, familiar terms. Analogies are popular in many subject areas. For instance, teachers commonly explain light in terms of particles and waves. But the instructor must fit the analogy to the new situation carefully; if the analogy does not fit, the student may develop misconceptions based on misapplications of the analogy. Implementing analogies in computerized instruction is also very easy.

Discovery- and hypothesis-testing learning strategies assume that a student can learn from the environment with little active help from the teacher. This approach recognizes that the mastery of a subject often requires the student to develop a series of hypotheses, and modify them as corroborating or disconfirming evidence is found. This learning strategy is particularly important in the development of techniques for medical diagnosis. To implement this strategy, a computer needs an internal model of the "real world" situation to provide diagnostic evidence to the students as they ask questions. The building of such computer models is difficult, and usually requires special programming.

LEARNING STRATEGIES AND CAI APPLICATIONS

Table 3

Learning Strategy	Examples of Use	Application Ease
Drill and Practice	Repetitive presentation of material; useful for learning of facts	Extremely easy for existing courseware authoring systems
Motivation	Use of gaming techniques to make lessons interesting	Could be difficult depending on techniques used
Learning by Example	Present example and then general rule	Easy for existing courseware authoring systems
Learning by Analogy	Relate new material to familiar knowledge	Easy for existing courseware authoring systems
Discovery and Hypothesis Testing	Unstructured; allows students to test hypotheses and discover knowledge on own	Not available in courseware authoring, must program
Spatial Problem Solving	Use of graphics to build up mental representation of task	Moderately easy if courseware authoring has graphics
Tutoring	Guides the students to the correct answers or strategies	Extremely difficult, no courseware authoring available

The cognitive skills of many experts are often based on spatial or geometric models. For example, an expert cardiologist may scan a mental image of a heart to match the patient's symptoms to a physical representation of possible causes. Graphics can help the student to construct such mental representations. The graphics capabilities of most courseware-authoring systems make it easy to write material for this learning strategy.

Tutoring—the specialized guidance of a student by a teacher—has long been beyond the capacity of computerized instruction. The teacher, unlike a computer, can respond precisely to student's open-ended questions within the context of voice inflexions, facial expressions, and the rapidity of the student's answers. Recently, natural-language processing has been applied to some CAI courses. But it is difficult to incorporate, and its success is still quite limited. Thus, tutoring is best done by humans.

In summary, the computer can be more effective than an instructor if teaching requires simulation models, graphics, or simple drill and practice.

REMAINING PROBLEMS

Computer-aided education systems have two major disadvantages. The first is the large time investment required to create a CAI course. Table 4 presents measures of the instructor time required to produce a single hour of instruction. The times reported vary considerably, depending on several factors. Some of the times were derived from controlled experimental data by recording the computer time required to compose the lessons. Others were simple author estimates, which are likely to be less accurate. Interestingly, the estimated times tend to be much lower than the experimental times, suggesting that authors often underestimate the amount of time they actually required to create their courses.

Author experience also influences the time it takes to create a course. Inexperienced authors require from 165 to 610 hours' work for each hour of computerized instruction. The nature of the authoring language is another influence. Course development using FORTRAN instead of a special authoring language required 2286

AUTHORING TIME*

Table 4

Hours per Hour of Instruction	Method of Estimation	Range or Type of Instruction	Experience of Author	Special Authoring Language?
2286	Averaged	Full	Not Specified	No
615	Averaged	Full	Not Specified	Yes
300	Estimate	Sophisticated	Inexperienced	Yes
295.1	Experiment Average	Full	Inexperienced	Yes
292	Averaged	Full	Inexperienced	Yes
250	Averaged	Simulation	Variable	Yes
200–500	Estimate	Sophisticated	Variable	Yes
196	Averaged	Full	Variable	Yes
165–610	Experiment Range	New Pedagogy	Low	Yes
151	Averaged	Full	Not Specified	Yes
100–150	Estimate	Comprehensive	Variable	Yes
82	Experiment	Moderate	High	Yes
80	Estimate	Full	High	Yes
72	Experiment	Moderate	High	Yes
54	Experiment	Moderate	High	Yes
49.7	Experiment Average	Moderate	Not Specified	Yes
32	Averaged	Full	Experienced	Yes
30–70	Estimate	Variable	Not Specified	Yes
27–180	Experiment Range	New Pedagogy	High	Yes
26.4	Experiment Average	Full	High	Yes
25–50	Estimate	Simple	Not Specified	Yes
22	Estimate	Simple	Not Specified	Yes
21	Estimate	Full	High	Yes
17	Experiment Average	Full	High	Yes
13	Experiment Average	Simple	Not Specified	Yes
8–63	Experiment Range	Existing Pedagogy	Low	Yes
8	Estimate	Not Specified	High	Yes
6.9	Experiment Average	Simple	Not Specified	Yes
6–39	Experiment Range	Simple	Low	Yes

*Full references can be found in [6].

hours' effort for a single hour of courseware! An authoring language is a far better choice if its capabilities fit the course material. Finally, the complexity of course material also plays a role in the time it takes to author a CAI lesson. Drill-and-practice lessons take less time to create than lessons that are simple variants of existing courses or pedagogies. A complete new course dealing with complicated material will take great amounts of time, as can be seen in Table 4.

A second problem is the unnaturalness of the computer interface. Students took twice as long to complete a computerized test as when taking the same test in paper-and-pencil form [13]. Learning how to use the computer seemed to consume the extra time. Another study [14] found that students took more time to make decisions when information was presented on a computer screen rather than on paper. Improvements in the computer/student interface are needed to make CAI techniques acceptable in all circumstances.

In both studies, the students had never used the particular computer system before. An initial time cost for learning to use a computer is always required. In other studies that showed a reduction in learning time when computers were used, the students had used the computers for many hours and had become comfortable with them. It should be possible to reduce the initial time needed to become comfortable with the computer.

REDUCTION IN AUTHORING TIME

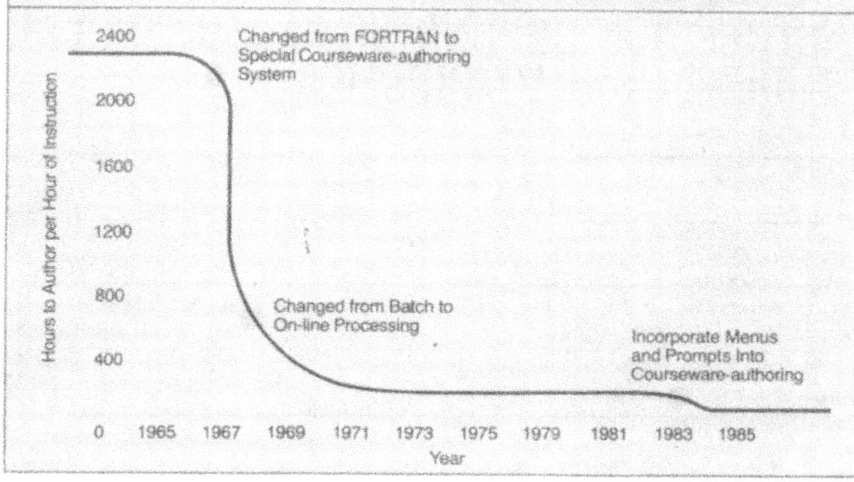

COMPUTERIZED EDUCATION IN THE FUTURE

Over the last twenty years, we have witnessed three major trends in computer-aided instruction: a reduction in authoring time; easier-to-use interfaces; and greater intelligence in the lesson presentation.

Figure 1 graphically shows how the time required to author a lesson has changed. Major milestones in this progress were the creation of authoring languages (instead of simple FORTRAN programs), conversion from batch-oriented to on-line interactive systems for authoring, and the development of authoring languages that employed menus and *help* screens. Continued improvements can be expected; and, as courseware becomes more available, authoring a course will more often be a matter of modifying existing courseware rather than starting from scratch.

Most current CAI systems require the student to interact with the keyboard. Touch screens and pointing devices (such as mice) are now available. Voice input devices are also available. Advances are being made by increasing the vocabulary such devices understand, and by making them speaker-independent.

Many have argued that CAI courses will not be able to compete with human-taught courses until the computer can understand natural language. But recent studies cast some doubt on the importance of a natural-language interface. Experiments have shown little difference in student performance whether natural-language interfaces or special query languages were used [15]. Furthermore, the natural-language interface may fool the student into thinking that the computer is smarter than it is, leading to mistakes and frustration when the student applies standard human-to-human communication techniques with the computer. The standard menu display should not be sold short, particularly when icon or touch-screen technology is employed. With intelligent design, students could ask open-ended questions by rearranging display symbols.

CAI programs are becoming more intelligent. Some research is focusing on tutoring methods that seek to guide the student to solutions without telling them exactly how to solve a problem. The secret of tutoring is knowing exactly when to interrupt the student's problem-solving activity—and knowing exactly what to say to that student.

Other researchers have taken a different tack. They have developed software that keeps an updated model of the knowledge of an individual student. The computer uses this model to decide what information to present or what other questions to ask the student. Such systems generally also contain an expert model of the course material. By comparing the student model with the expert model, the systems decide what information to provide the student in order to transform him into an expert efficiently. These more intelligent systems may reduce the total authoring effort. Presently, courseware authors must predict all of the students' possible responses to each question in the lesson, and develop explicit lesson pathways for each response. With the above modeling techniques, it is possible that the computer could generate the expected lesson pathways as well as unexpected ones, without explicit author effort.

The future of computerized instruction looks promising. Already, much courseware exists; CAI may save student time, and the computer cost of providing an hour of CAI instruction is competitive with the cost of human lecture time. For computerization to reach its full potential, the burden of authoring time must be greatly reduced, and student/computer interactions made easier. The quality of a CAI course depends just as much upon the author's energy, effort, and imagination as does a comparable lecture or textbook. The computer will not salvage mediocre course material any more than television would improve the impact of a poor lecture. CAI has great potential in postgraduate and continuing medical education because of the quantity of material, and because so much is suitable for drill and practice or modeling. But teachers must have a strong role in the development of this tool if it is to achieve its promise. □

ONE GOAL OF COMPUTER-AIDED EDUCATION HAS BEEN TO CHANGE INSTRUCTION DEPENDING ON PARTICULAR STUDENT CHARACTERISTICS.

REFERENCES

1. Bunderson CV. Courseware. In: O'Neil HF, ed. Computer-based instruction: a state-of-the-art assessment. New York: Academic Press, 1981:91–125.

2. Kearsley GP. Authoring tools: An introduction. J Comput-Based Instr 1984; 11:67.

3. Mace T. Education. In: Annual software review. PC World 1985; 2(14):254–70.

4. Eberts RE. Learning strategies and CAI design. In: Grayson LP, Biedenbach JM, ed. Computer aided engineering. Washington, DC: American Society for Engineering Education, 1985:791–7.

5. Hofstetter FT. The cost of PLATO in a university environment. J Comput-Based Instr 1983; 9:248–55.

6. Eberts RE, Brock JB. Computer assisted and computer managed instruction. In: Salvendy G, ed. Human factors handbook. New York: John Wiley, 1986 (forthcoming).

7. Conkwright TD. PLATO applications in the airline industry. J Comput-Based Instr 1982; 8:49–52.

8. Orlansky J, String J. Cost-effectiveness of computer-based instruction in military training. IDA Paper P-1375. Arlington, VA: Institute for Defense Analyses, 1977.

9. Morgan CE. CAI and basic skills information. Ed Tech 1978; 18(4):37–9.

10. Avner A, Moore C, Smith S. CBI authoring tools: effects on productivity and quality. J Comput-Based Instr 1984; 11:85–9.

11. Buck JA. Federal Aviation Administration seventh year computer-based training report. J Comput-Based Instr 1982; 8:53–5.

12. Montague WE, Wulfeck WH, Ellis JA. Quality CAI depends on quality instructional design and quality implementation. J Comput-Based Instr 1980; 10:90–3.

13. Hansen WJ, Doring R, Whitlock LR. Why an examination was slower on-line than on paper. Int J Man-Machine Studies 1978; 10:507–19.

14. Kozar KA, Dickson GW. An experimental study of the effects of data display media on decision effectiveness. Int J Man-Machine Studies 1978; 10:495–505.

15. Small DW, Weldon LJ. An experimental comparison of natural and structured query languages. Hum Factors 1983; 25:253–63.

PRODUCT INFORMATION

For further information about medical education programs at Massachusetts General Hospital:

- Minet Medical Information Network for GTE Telenet:

Medical Information Network
8229 Boone Boulevard
Vienna, VA 22180
800/368-4215

- For microcomputers:

CPR Training by Computer
Williams and Wilkins
Electronic Media Division
428 E. Preston Street
Baltimore, MD 21202
800/638-0672
$85 for the complete program.

For information about medical education programs at the University of Seattle:

- Clinical Patient Simulation

CME Incorporated
P.O. Box 85655
University Station
Seattle, WA 98145-1655
206/524-0298
24 different cases are available at various prices.

TALK IS GETTING CHEAP

STEVEN M. AND LYNN ENTINE

Everybody's talking at you, and chances are the voices are not human. They are coming from your car, the telephone, your vending machine, and your microcomputer. Computerized speech generation has arrived. Though your home or office microcomputer will not replace C3PO's part in the next *Star Wars* film, it is potentially useful at home, in the office, lab, examining room, or hospital.

STEVEN AND LYNN ENTINE

Steven M. Entine is Project Supervisor in charge of data management at the Wisconsin Clinical Cancer Center, University of Wisconsin-Madison. He has been analyzing and designing computer systems for more than twenty years, ten years in medical applications. His work has included database management, patient simulations and speech technology. Lynn Entine is a professional writer who has more than three dozen published articles and pamphlets to her credit. She specializes in writing about science and business. When they are not busy collaborating on writing projects they put their energies into keeping up with their three-year-old daughter.

Speech generation is only one half of the new voice technology—the more advanced half. The other is speech recognition, where a computer "hears" and responds to verbal commands. Some of these systems already operate effectively, especially as handicap aids. One long-term goal of speech recognition technology is to provide printed text directly from spoken input. Pathologists doing postmortems, or laboratory technicians whose hands and eyes are busy, could generate reports directly and quickly. This article introduces the current status of speech generation and recognition technology and describes current and future medical applications.

SPEECH GENERATION: HOW IT WORKS

Two technologies generate speech output: digital storage of spoken words or phrases, and synthetic generation of words from stored phonemes (basic units of speech). The first has the potential for producing high-quality output on a predefined vocabulary. The second permits voice output of an unlimited number of words.

DIGITALLY STORED SPEECH

AT&T pioneered digitized speech for long-distance telephone calls. The simplest digitizing technique, pulse code modulation, requires sampling the strength of the speech signal 8,000 times per second. Each sample is assigned a number from 0 to 255 [1]. The stream of digits flows through digital to analog circuitry to reproduce the sound up to 4,000 Hz (cycles per second), an adequate range for the human voice. (A typical stereo amplifier responds to frequencies up to 20,000 Hz, so you will not be playing symphonies on your computer.) Pulse code modulation requires 8,000 bytes of data per second. Thus, a typical floppy disk for a microcomputer could hold only about 140 words, or the equivalent of 40 seconds of speech.

This large storage requirement spurred research into discovering ways of compressing the speech signal into a smaller number of bytes. One method, continuous variable-slope delta modulation, reduces the storage rate for speech from 8,000 bytes per second to approximately 1,500 bytes per second [2].

Another compression technique is linear predictive coding (LPC). This reduces the data rate to approximately 150 bytes per second. To achieve this, the signal is split into different frequency ranges and each of these is sampled. The results then become data for a mathematical model of the vocal tract. This reduction requires complex computations at the time words are stored and again when the recorded coefficients are used to generate speech. It grew popular after Texas Instruments introduced a single chip LPC speech synthesizer which drastically lowered costs for producing speech from stored LPC data. However, development machines, which permit users to build their own vocabulary, still cost $29,000–35,000 [2].

The advantage of digitally stored speech is its good quality of voice output. When a voice on a telephone line announces: "The number you have reached has been changed; the new number is 555–9416," almost everyone can understand it, despite the unnatural pauses between numbers.

RULE-GENERATED SPEECH

The other technique for generating speech output uses rules for synthesizing it. Speech is broken into units smaller than individual words, ranging in size from phonemes (the basic sounds of all speech) to parts of syllables. Information on how to generate sound from each stored unit is normally contained within special-purpose hardware. For a word to be spoken, the appropriate sequence of stored units must be triggered. The major work in this area is in devising complex linguistic rules describing how to translate from the spelling of a word to the appropriate sequence of sounds. These rules are then programmed on the microprocessor contained in the speech synthesizer. Producing verbal rather than printed output in application programs is a simple process of selecting an alternative communication channel.

The quality of output from rule-originated speech synthesis varies from very poor to tolerable. The Votrax "Type and Talk" ($249) generates words with an accuracy of recognition rate of 65–70% by untrained users [1]. The Prose 2,000 by Speech Plus ($4800) can satisfactorily speak a customer name and address list [2]. The difference between the two is sophistication in the rules. Lower-quality systems may require users to utilize "creative" spelling in order to achieve acceptable output. This can lead to keeping dual file systems—one with correct spellings for printing and a second with spellings for speech.

The human brain collects much of its information about language from inflection, emphasis, and varied pronunciations which change with both meaning and context. For example, the final "g" in words ending in "-ing" is often dropped when another word follows it. "I'll be seeing you" when spoken typically sounds more like "Ahl b'seen ya." Synthetic speech, whether digitized or rule-generated, produces something like:

I
'll
bee
see
ing
you

Some of this linguistic variability has been codified and included in the more sophisticated rules. Much of it is still unquantified.

A second problem shared by both types of voice output is that each generates discrete words. Putting them together into meaningful sentences requires an additional set of rules regarding emphasis and inflection. The systems must be taught to indicate a question with a rising intonation at the end of a sentence. Variance in meaning resulting from selective word emphasis is beyond their capability. The difference in meanings, for example, between "What are *you* doing here?" and "What are you *doing* here?" is lost in computerized speech generation.

Because the computer's voice is alien and may be difficult to understand, it is tiring to listen to it for more than a few minutes. "Speech," explains Ron Carlson, principal engineer of Mattell Electronics in Hawthorne, California, "is normally a function interpreted by Broca's area in the left brain. If speech begins to get unintelligible, the brain starts dividing its attention between parsing the speech and figuring out what it heard, which emerges as a competing task. If speech gets too unintelligible, the right hemisphere of the brain takes over and starts to interpret what it hears almost as music, responding to the pattern and the rhythm of the sound instead of to its content. Some speech systems are so unintelligible that an innocent listener isn't even sure it's speech. And it doesn't take very many competing tasks before the intelligibility becomes unacceptable" [3].

The quality required of voice output depends on its use. Where a few words are used repeatedly, as in voice prompts for data input for example, low quality is offset by user familiarity and limited length of continuous listening time. In text-to-speech applications such as the Kurzweil reading machine for the blind, much higher quality is important for comprehension and listener endurance. The potential for distraction from computer-generated speech becomes an important consideration in high-stress situations where computer assistance might be a benefit, such as ICUs and emergency rooms.

MEDICAL USES FOR VOICE OUTPUT

The most well developed application of computer voice output is in aids to the handicapped. The Kurzweil reader has opened literally millions of volumes of material to the blind. In addition, speakers attached to computers announce each letter as it is entered by a blind person, improving input accuracy tremendously. This opens data entry and processing jobs to the visually handicapped. Vocally handicapped persons can use computer synthesized speech to communicate for them over the phone and in person.

Currently available technology makes it possible to use voice output in alerting devices. ICU monitors might follow a buzzer with a statement like "Bed 3, heart arrythmia." This would help ICU staff anticipate what instruments or medications to take with them on the way to check the patient.

Computer monitors on labora-

SPEECH GENERATION DEVICES

COMPANY	DEVICE	COST ($)	COMPUTER	TYPE
Allen Group 27 West 23rd Street New York, NY 10010	Voice Box	$ 169.00 215.00 95.00	Atari 400, 800 Apple II, II+, IIe Commodore VIC-20	Hardware Hardware Hardware
Centigram Corp. 1362 Borregas Avenue Sunnyvale, CA 94087	SYBIL	495.00	IBM PC	Hardware
Commodore 1200 Wilson Drive West Chester, PA 19380	Speech Module	?	Commodore 64	Hardware
Intex Micro Systems 725 S. Adams Road Birmingham, MI 48011	Intex-Talker	295.00	RS-232 port Centronics (parallel port)	Hardware
Maintain Computer 300 El Pueblo Road Scotts Valley, CA 95066	Supertalker II SD200	565.00 199.00	IBM-PC Apple II, IIe	Hardware Hardware
Soft Tape 5547 Satsuma Avenue N. Hollywood, CA 91601	Apple Talk	29.95	Apple II, II+, IIe	Software
Speech Plus, Inc. 461 N. Bernardo Avenue Mountain View, CA 94043	Speech 1000 Speech 1020 Prose 2000 Prose 2020	$1200 + vocab 2500 + vocab 3500 4800	RS-232 RS-232 RS-232 RS-232	Hardware Hardware Hardware Hardware
Street Electronics 1140 Mark Avenue Carpenteria, CA 93013	Echo II Echo GP	149.95 299.95	Apple II RS-232	Hardware Hardware
Telesensory Systems, Inc. 455 North Bernardo Avenue Mountain View, CA 94043	VERT 6000	5995.00 +495.00	RS-232	Hardware Software
Texas Instruments Box 53 Lubbock, TX 79408	Speech Synthesizer	99.95	TI 99/4A	Hardware
Votrax 500 Stephenson Highway Troy, MI 48084	Personal Speech System Type-N-Talk	395.00 249.00	RS-232 (serial port) Centronics (parallel port) RS-232	Hardware Hardware
Vynet Corp. 160B Albright Way Los Gatos, CA 95030	V200-USM	444.00	Apple II, II+, IIe IBM-PC	Info not available

tory equipment could announce completion of a long-running test; malfunction of freezers, heaters, and the like; problems such as paper jams on printers; temperature variations and even fire, or entry of burglars. Particularly when coupled with an automatic telephone dialing device, voice description of problems in alerting situations can save time and improve efficiency of response.

Remote access to computers without a terminal is another application of voice output. A physician can use a touch-tone telephone and immediately receive information on the next day's clinic schedule or obtain results from the clinical laboratory. This would open up the use of hospital information systems or clinical management systems to physicians when they are at meetings or other locations where telephones are common but terminals inaccessible.

THE BEST-DEVELOPED VOICE OUTPUT APPLICATIONS ARE AIDS FOR THE HANDICAPPED. THE KURZWEIL READER HAS OPENED COUNTLESS BOOKS TO THE BLIND.

In the future, national information networks may be accessible from touch-tone telephones. Access to systems such as MEDLINE will improve their utility and flexibility. A researcher could enter a billing code by touchtone, and then be guided through a branching system of keywords making touchtone responses. The user would then hear citations of selected articles. (When voice output can be coupled with voice recognition, the researcher could speak the keywords rather than using the limited responses available on the touchtone pad.)

Wherever computers are used, whether in medical teaching situations, clinic and hospital offices, or when patients interact directly with computers, voice explanations of prompts could help the user who may be having difficulty understanding how to work the terminal or computer keyboard. A significant delay in responding to a visual prompt might, for example, cue the computer to repeat the prompt with additional information such as "When you enter your sex, type F or M, then the escape key. The escape key is labeled e-s-c and is located in the upper left corner of the keyboard."

There are dozens of potential uses for computerized speech output. However, both existing voice output techniques are tiring to listen to because sentences are constructed of discrete words and lack information normally conveyed by inflection, intonation, and emphasis. For highly motivated users such as the visually or vocally handicapped, voice output devices are already very useful. Their utility in other situations will depend on the motivation of the user, and the relative availability of alternatives.

SPEECH RECOGNITION

People communicate most easily with spoken words. Speech is more universal than reading, and faster than writing or typing. So it is natural that both in fantasy and reality people want to talk to computers. From the earliest robots envisioned by Asimov through *Star Trek*, *2001*, and *Star Wars* everybody talks to computers. Technology, however, lags far behind fantasy.

Speech recognition technology must solve two general problems: speaker dependency and continuous speech recognition. Speaker-dependent systems require each user to train the system. They cannot respond to words spoken by any casual visitor. Speaker-independent systems are unrestricted. Discrete recognition systems require users to make a clean pause between any two words, while continuous recognition permits users to speak in a normal conversational flow.

Most current systems are speaker dependent and discrete. They recognize words through a "training" program which must be used by each operator. Depending on the specific system, the speaker records each word from two to ten times using a microphone input to the system. In addition, the user must also specify what information the computer is to send the operating program when it recognizes a verbal command. The computer analyzes these digital speech records for similarities and differences and saves an "average" pronunciation. Variations that are too great cause it to reject the entire sample. (This eliminates problems with extraneous noises like sneezes, telephone bells, etc.) Minor variations in tone, inflection, and pitch are saved within the template or pattern. These templates are formed by using technology, such as power-spectral density, where the signal is split into different frequency ranges and the strength of each of these is sampled. Since this produces a large amount of data, recognition systems require a large amount of both processor power and storage.

Once a dictionary of templates and "words" is defined, the system can be used for voice recognition. When the device "hears" a word spoken, it digitally records it, then compares the new word template with each template in its dictionary. When the word is found, it transmits an associated command to the operating program. A voice recognition system of this type helps Robbie Marince, a quadraplegic man. He uses it to control his television and other devices in his home. He is able to go to school, run a Betamax to review his lessons, answer the telephone and make telephone calls—all by voice control [4].

There are several disadvantages to this technology. For one, the system's use is limited to a single person although it may be expanded to several users if each of them first "trains" the computer in his or her particular speech patterns. As the size of the vocabulary and number of intended users increases, this restriction becomes more critical. When staff are large or turnover is frequent the expense of "training" the computer may become prohibitive, particularly if technology should permit vocabularies of thousands of words. Of course, in some applications, speaker dependency can be a security advantage. A physician giving clinical orders by voice could not be impersonated, even by someone as convincing as Rich Little, since voice patterns are as unique to individuals as fingerprints.

The second disadvantage is the large amount of storage required for each template. This restricts the vocabulary size of recognition systems. A related problem is the method used by the computer to recognize a spoken word. Since there is no logic available to help it search, it must compare the input word to each item in its vocabulary in turn. Thus, the more words it "knows," the longer it takes to respond. This problem limits not only the vocabulary but also the number of speakers (i.e.,

10 speakers with 100 words equals a 1,000 word vocabulary).

Some systems, such as the Plessey, permit users to activate a limited (100–200-word) vocabulary from a larger dictionary which is stored off-line on the disk of the host computer. Thus, in a system with 10 users, each one could identify his or her own set of 100–200 templates stored on the disk and could call them up when signing on.

An additional problem with the template technology arises from the similarity of sounds and words in English. The letters *b*, *c*, *d*, *e*, *g*, *p*, *t*, *v*, and *z* are so similar that their digital templates can be difficult if not impossible to distinguish. Most current systems cannot successfully distinguish the letters of the alphabet at an acceptable error rate.

Words that sound alike pose a similar problem; e.g., bee, tea, pea; thing, sling, sting. Systems are far more accurate when the words in their dictionary sound quite distinct from one another. Performance ratings for systems should ideally include the actual words used for the test.

Reliance on the use of discrete words in speech recognition systems is also a disadvantage. In order for the computer to recognize and respond to a command, the speaker must surround it with silence. The wait between words can vary significantly between systems. A requirement for lengthy pauses quickly becomes tiring and distracting to the user.

Even with current technology in its infancy, voice recognition systems are finding applications. The Tecmar system has a 100-word vocabulary with 98 percent accuracy. Its uses are primarily in activating other system components for users whose hands are occupied or incapable of performing the function. One application of their system is to couple speech recognition with conventional voice technology, such as dictation units and voice mail (a system which encodes and files voice messages on a disk for transmission, much as electronic mail transmits written messages).

As with the speech generation applications, the advantage of recognition is remote operation without a terminal. In one example, a physician at a hospital office could telephone to an automatic dictation unit, turn it on with a command such as "dictate on," dictate a letter, and command it to be sent to a different location such as a clinic office, where it could be transcribed. When the physician arrives at the clinic office the final document is ready for signature.

SPEECH RECOGNITION SYSTEMS

MANUFACTURER	MODEL	VOCABULARY	COST
Heuristics System 1285 Hammerwood Avenue Sunnyvale, CA 94086	Model 7000	64 to 128 words	$3000
Keytronic Voice Input Device P.O. Box 14687 Spokane, VA 99214		100 words	$1200
Interstate Electronics Corporation 1001 E. Ball Rd. P.O. Box 3117 Anaheim, CA 92803	VRM	100 words	$2255
NEC America, Inc. 532 Broad Hollow Road Melville, NY 11747	DP-100 DP-200	50 to 500 words	$12,000
Plessy Peripheral Systems Inc. 2632 Du-Bridge Avenue Irvine, CA 92714	PVRT 300	100 words	$1300
Techmar Voice Recognition 2360 Mercantile Road Cleveland, OH 44122		100 to 2000 words	$995
Votan 4487 Technology Drive Freemont, CA 94538	V-8000	255 words	$9000

SPEAKER-INDEPENDENT AND CONTINUOUS SPEECH SYSTEMS

If you have ever listened to somebody's two-year-old proudly demonstrating verbal skills, and found the child to be totally unintelligible, you have a sense of the problems facing speaker-independent speech recognition systems. Systems developed for a speaker from the South would need additional tools to respond also to a Brooklyn accent. Non-native speakers of English would probably be excluded because of their accents. Currently there are no speaker-independent small-scale systems ready for production use. A few systems that can recognize a small vocabulary of words are available, but these require large computers with extensive memories and processing capability.

One specialist, Ronald Cole of Carnegie-Mellon's speech recognition laboratory, predicts that within two to three years speaker-independent speech recognition of digits and small vocabularies (10–30 words) will be available for under $100 [4]. Digit recognition will be useful for accounting tasks, voice dialing of telephones, and paging systems.

Continuous speech recognition technology is farther in the future. The technology required for such systems, feature-based recognition, is similar to speech synthesis by rule. Instead of storing templates for each word or each sound and then matching each spoken word with the templates in its dictionary, this system identifies words by identifying their phonetic components. According to Cole: "It'd be like saying 'an "s" sound has high-frequency noise and it's so long' or 'a "p" sound has silence, and then it has an abrupt onset,' and so forth" [4]. Rather than storing a template, this technology requires only that descriptions of phonetic features, one or more phonetic spellings, and the desired text or command be kept in the dictionary for each word. This would result in a drastic reduction in the storage required. When it becomes available, the feature-based recognition system will be speaker-independent, have large vocabularies, and be much faster and more flexible because it can use rules for searching rather than matching templates.

As with the template technology, feature recognition is hampered by the complexity of language and phonetic similarities. Minor variations in words change the meaning without significantly altering the sound: feet, fleet, sleet, seat, etc. Homonyms and puns are additional challenges. Consider a speech recognition system sorting out "bear" and "bare"; "two," "too," and "to." In a continuous stream of speech, divisions between words often are lost. For example, consider the ambiguity between "chair and table" and "charitable." In languages such as Chinese, which rely on tone level as well as pronunciation for meaning, the problems are even more difficult.

The proof that speech recognition systems are feasible and useful would be the development of an automatic dictation machine that can recognize words in the continuous flow of speech, use meaning to distinguish between the various phonetic segments, and use intonation and pace to punctuate the text correctly [4]. Translating speech directly to text without a human transcriber will then be fast and efficient—a revolution comparable to the introduction of VDTs to newspaper and magazine publishing.

Such a revolution is decades in the future. Research in language recognition has taken two separate paths, both complex, and both needing resolution before automatic dictation equipment is feasible. Computer artificial intelligence research is making some progress in understanding "natural language" (as opposed to the stylized forms traditionally required by computers). This work centers on standard keyboard entry of information.

The most promising continuous speech recognition research focuses on isolating individual words from the continuous speech flow, using complex rules for variations in word pronunciation within the context of a sentence. Once words can be identified as individual entities, grammar rules and other information can be used to restrict the number of possible dictionary entries to which each must be matched. Some sounds are sufficiently unique that the number of possible words to which they belong is very small. Even with breakthroughs in both these areas, it is unrealistic to expect that computers will be able to do a more accurate job than human transcribers in understanding unfamiliar names, distinguishing between homonyms, and correctly interpreting dictated messages among background noises, throat clearings, and other extraneous sound.

SUMMARY

In summary, computer speech is currently generated by two technologies: digitally stored speech and rule-generated speech. Digitally stored speech is most easily understood; however, it requires relatively large amounts of memory space and special equipment to enter speech into memory. Digital speech storage systems have a limited vocabulary, and it is not easy for users to expand or alter it.

Rule-generated speech is less easily understood than digital speech. Quality varies depending on the sophistication and cost of the speech-synthesizing device. The functional vocabulary for rule-generated speech is unlimited. Some systems now available contain both technologies. However, any one application would best be confined to a single technology, since the user would likely be quite distracted by the noticeable shifts in voice quality between the two systems.

Speech recognition technology lags far behind speech generation. It is significantly more complex. Speech generators produce a precise, consistent signal and send it to a highly intelligent and flexible receiver—the human ear and brain. In speech recognition, a highly complex and variable signal (human speech) is being sent to a limited and relatively inflexible receiver (the computer program). In the near future, development of speech recognition technology will occur in two areas. As the speed of microprocessors and special circuitry increases, and as memory prices decrease, the vocabulary size in speaker-dependent systems will increase. Second, speaker-independent systems with extremely limited vocabularies will become widely available. While work will continue in feature recognition, systems capable of understanding large vocabularies remain years away. It will be a long time before computers will be able to laugh at your puns.

SELECTING A DISPLAY MONITOR

RICHARD FRIEDMAN, M.D.

The monitor is the principal communications link between microcomputer and user. Yet it is virtually ignored by most purchasers, who merely accept the vendor's bundled display device. The bundled monitors are quite acceptable, given the advantages of compatibility and one-vendor service support. But it can pay to shop around for a monitor, particularly if you are interested in a low-cost monochrome display device (a good monochrome device can be obtained for under $100), a high-resolution RGB (Red Green Blue) color monitor, or one with specialized capabilities (such as touch screen, large screen, or specialized graphics controller).

RICHARD B. FRIEDMAN, M.D.
Dr. Friedman is an Associate Professor of Medicine and Head of the General Internal Medicine Section at the University of Wisconsin Medical School. He is a practicing internist with research interests in the application of computers to medical education and clinical competence evaluation. He also has published papers in the area of clinical laboratory automation.

Dr. Friedman has been working with computers since 1960, when he programmed Columbia University's IBM 650. When not doctoring or computing he is sailing.

All monitors that you can buy as separate devices are currently based on cathode ray tube (CRT) technology. The image on a CRT appears when electrons from the CRT electron gun excite the phosphor on the inner side of the glass, causing it to emit photons. The unexcited portion remains dark to provide the background. (In a reverse video display, the background is excited and the image remains dark, to give the look of a printed page.) The beam moves downward, painting lines from left to right. (On some monitors, during a second sweep, the beam paints intermediate lines.) Monochrome monitors use a continuous phosphor coating; color monitors use triads of dots or vertical stripes of different inorganic phosphors. One dot (or stripe) emits red light when excited, one emits blue, and one emits green. Combinations of these make the different colors.

There are four different types of CRT monitors. The simplest is the standard television set. To use it requires a radio-frequency (RF) modulator (which can cost less than $10) to convert the computer-generated signals into a format the TV set can understand. The major limitations of this type of display are its mediocre color and resolution and its low maximum output (40 characters per line).

The most common type of microcomputer display device is the monochrome monitor. This monitor displays 80 characters per line but in one color—usually green, white, or amber—on black. Monochrome monitors generally print text that is crisper than that of color monitors, and thus are preferred for text manipulation. Monochrome can also produce higher-resolution graphics than color, with the right signal generation. Special monochrome boards, like the Hercules, can simultaneously display text and graphics, while the IBM monochrome board is limited to the display of one or the other. The Hercules board is widely supported by popular products, such as MicroSoft Word and Lotus 1-2-3.

A composite video color (CVC) monitor is like a TV set in that it accepts direct video input. It produces a better image than does the RF-modulated color TV. (In the RF conversion, part of the original signal is lost, and unwanted video "noise" can enter the signal.) Con-

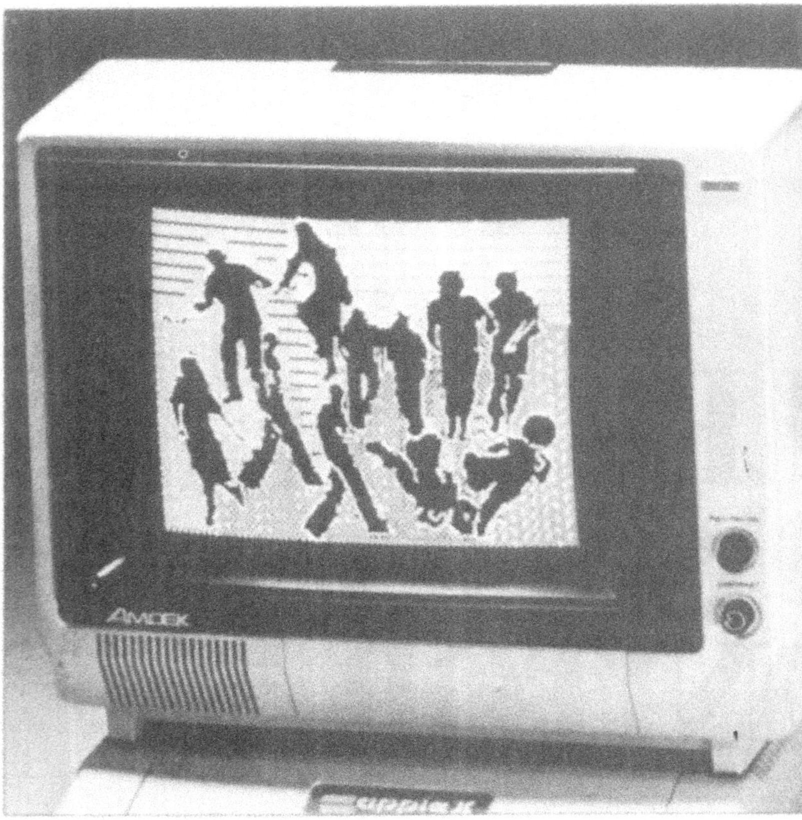

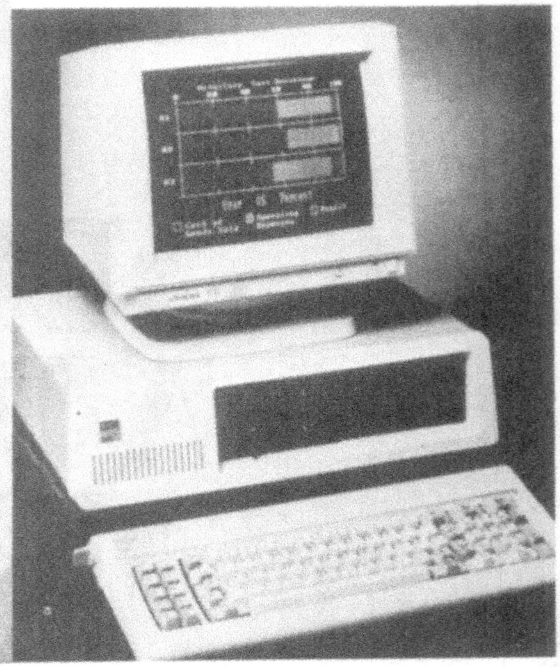

forming to National Television Standards Committee (NTSC) standards, a composite video monitor accepts black-and-white and color (red, green, and blue), horizontal and vertical synchronization information in one signal. A composite monitor uses three separate electron guns (one for each primary color). The color is not as sharp as that produced by the red-green-blue (RGB) monitor (described next) because information in this signal has a limited bandwidth, which must be decoded by synchronous demodulators with their attendant phase and gain problems. What is worse, the output usually has the same 40-character output limits as a TV set monitor.

An RGB monitor provides the best color image. Its superiority is due to its use of *three* separate input signals (one for each "primary" color), with horizontal and vertical synchronization transmitted as a separate signal or superimposed on one of the three color signals—usually green. As in composite video, each color signal is fed to a separate electron gun which is slightly angled. The angle of the gun and the use of a shadow mask permit each beam to strike the proper phosphor dot or stripe. There are two types of RGB signals. Analog RGB permits the level of each color to be varied continuously to yield an infinite variety of brightness levels and colors. Transitor-transitor logic (TTL) RGB uses a simpler logic, with each of the color signals being either on or off at any time. Because there is no single RGB standard, you must be sure about monitor/microcomputer compatibility before buying an RGB monitor. Try the monitor with your computer before buying.

In addition to these four basic types of CRT monitors, newer technologies have been adapted for use in display devices, including gas plasma monitors and liquid crystal display. All of these have the advantage of flatness, low weight, and less bulk than a CRT.

Gas plasma monitors use ionized gas sandwiched between two glass plates lined with a series of parallel horizontal and vertical wires. When current is sent to an intersection of wires, the gas at that point produces a dot of orange light. Plasma monitors have the advantage of very high resolution (960 pixels horizontal 768 vertical on the IBM 581 monitor), absence of glare and flicker, and easy viewing from all angles. The IBM

Modern monitors can produce a wide variety of graphics when operated through a personal computer. Two RGB color monitors are pictured above: the Amdek Color-I (left) and the Amdek Color 710 (right).

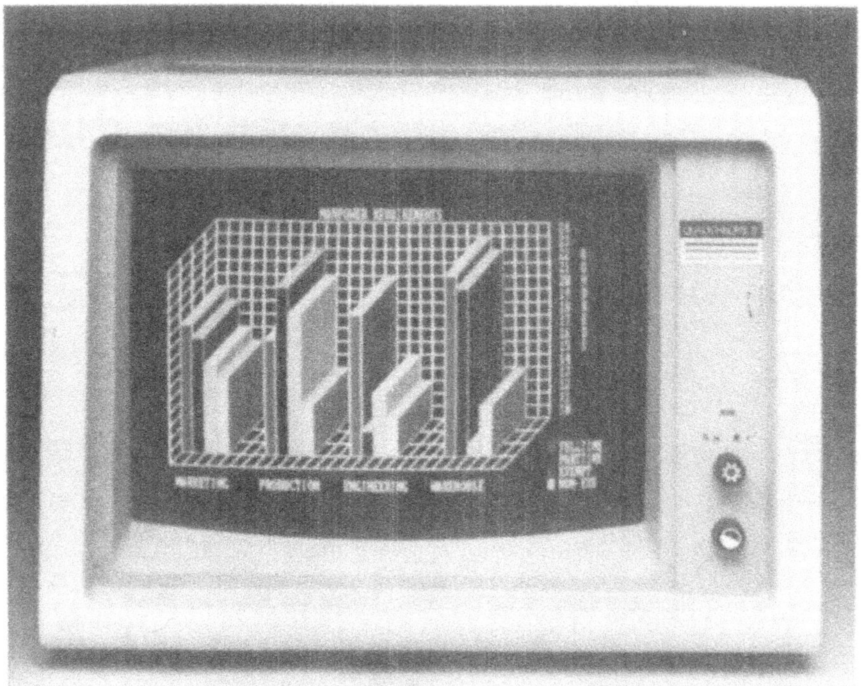

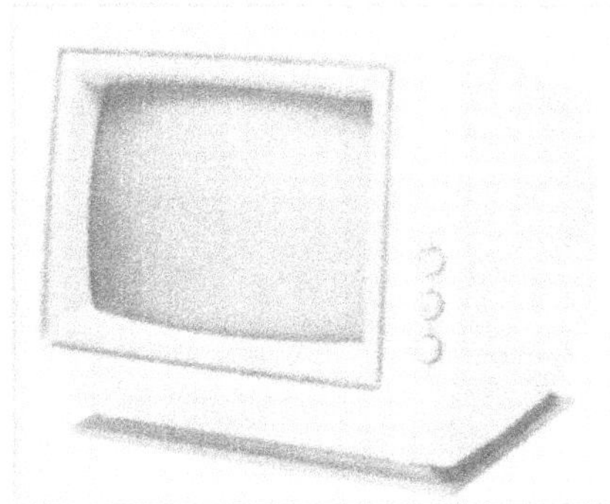

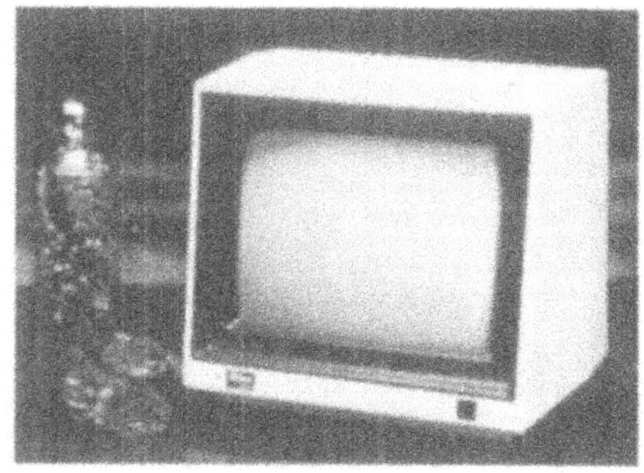

More examples of high-resolution monitors: the color Quadchrome II by Quadram (above left) and Sanyo's monochrome DM 9112 (upper right). Among the features of Sakata's SC-100 CRT composite color display monitor (lower right) is a phone jack for sound output.

display can present 69 lines, each with 180 characters. Most importantly, gas plasma displays are flat panels—not bulky boxes containing large tubes. The major drawbacks of such displays are their cost (the IBM gas plasma display is $3,000), their color (only a glaring orange) and their voltage, which is too high to permit use in portable machines. However, their high resolution permits very large displays, and the price is expected to drop.

Liquid crystal displays (LCDs) draw very little current. They are found in most battery-powered portable computers. The most widely available LCDs on computers provide only 8 lines of 24 characters. But displays offering 16 lines of 80 characters are available, and displays of 24 lines of 80 characters are ready for commercialization. Because these displays are relatively low in cost and require little voltage, they are ideal for portable applications. They have disadvantages, however. Like digital watches, they can be read only from a narrow viewing angle, and they cannot be read in low light. In addition, their painting time is relatively slow. However, only LCD's have the potential for competing with the cost of the conventional CRT.

There are other technologies, such as electroluminescent display, electrophoretic displays, and vacuum fluorescence, which have great promise but are not as well developed as those mentioned above. A thorough but quite readable review of flat-panel technology is given in Reference 1.

Flat-panel technology has immediate relevance only to portable computers. For day-in and day-out use, a standard CRT cannot be beat. Let us look at the characteristics to consider when reviewing CRT monitors for purchase.

MONITOR CHARACTERISTICS

Diagonal Display Size

This is the measure across the diagonal of the screen. As this measurement increases, either more information can be displayed (using a column with more than 80 characters) or a larger character matrix can be used. The most common diagonal display size is 12 or 13 inches, but larger sizes (15-, 17-, and 25-inch displays) are now available.

Character Display

Most monitors display 24 or 25 lines of 80 characters each. However, television sets and composite

SELECTED MONOCHROME MONITORS

Table 1

MANUFACTURER AND MODELS	DIAGONAL SIZE (INCHES)	DISPLAY CAPACITY: LINES	DISPLAY CAPACITY: CHARACTERS	CHARACTER MATRIX (DOTS)	RESOLUTION (PIXELS)†	COLOR	COMPATIBLE WITH: APPLE II?	COMPATIBLE WITH: IBM-PC?	COST
Amdek									
Video 300	12	24	80	5 × 7	960	Green	Yes	Yes	$ 179
						Amber	Yes	Yes	$ 199
Video 310 A	12	24	80	5 × 7	960	Amber	No	Yes	$ 230
Apple Computers									
Apple II	12	24	80	5 × 7	900	Green	Yes	Yes	$ 229
Apple III	12	24	80	5 × 7	700	Green	Yes	Yes	$ 249
Comrex International Inc.									
CR-5400	9	25	132	5 × 7	650 × 240	Green	Yes	Yes	$ 149
						Amber	Yes	Yes	$ 159
CR-5600	12	25	132	5 × 7	1000 × 240	Green	Yes	Yes	$ 169
						Amber	Yes	Yes	$ 189
Dynax									
AM 121	12	25	80	N/A*	600	Amber	Yes	Yes	$ 219
GM 120	12	25	80	N/A	600	Green	Yes	Yes	$ 199
Hitachi America									
MM 1218	12	24	80	7 × 9 9 × 14	N/A	Green	Yes	Yes	$ 223
IBM (Systems Products Division)									
Monochrome	11.5	25	80		720 × 350	Green	No	Yes	$ 345
Leading Edge Products, Inc.									
Gorilla	12	25	80	5 × 7	850 × 245	Green	Yes	Yes	$ 99
						Amber	Yes	Yes	$ 104
Genius Model 102	15	57	80	9 × 14	720 × 800	Green	Yes	Yes	$1395
						Amber	Yes	Yes	$1395
NEC Home Electronics (Personal Computer Division)									
JB-1260 MA	12	25	80	8 × 8	600 × 230	Green	Yes	Yes	$ 149
JB-1201 MA	12	25	80	8 × 8	800 × 230	Green	Yes	Yes	$ 199
JB-902A	9	25	80	8 × 8	700 × 230	Green	Yes	Yes	$ 189
JB-1205MA	12	25	80	8 × 8	800 × 230	Amber	Yes	Yes	$ 210
Princeton Graphic Systems									
Max-12	12	25	80	9 × 14	720 × 350	Amber	No	Yes	$ 249
Quadram Corp.									
Quadscreen	17	25	80	5 × 7, 11 × 9	960 × 512	White	No	Yes	$1995
Sakata U.S.A. Corporation									
SC-1000	12	25	80	5 × 7	900	Green	Yes	Yes	$ 129
Sanyo Electric									
DM 2112/2212	12	25	64	5 × 7	340 × 230	Green	Yes	Yes	$ 145
						Amber	Yes	Yes	$ 145
DM 8012/ 8112/8212	12	25	80	5 × 7	480 × 240	Green	Yes	Yes	$ 240
						Amber	Yes	Yes	$ 240
DM 9012/ 9112/9212	12	25	80	5 × 7	480 × 240	Green	Yes	Yes	$ 260
						Amber	Yes	Yes	$ 260
USI Computer Products									
P11	9	25	80	5 × 7	1000	Green	Yes	Yes	$ 159
P12	12	25	80	5 × 7	1000	Green	Yes	Yes	$ 199
P13	12	25	80	5 × 7	1000	Amber	Yes	Yes	$ 239
P14	9	25	80	5 × 7	1000	Amber	Yes	Yes	$ 199
Zenith Electronics Corp. (Zenith Data Systems Division)									
ZVM124	12	25	80	7 × 9	900	Amber	Yes	No	$ 199

* N/A = Information not available.
† Where only one number is given, it represents the number of pixels across a horizontal line.

SELECTED RGB MONITORS

Table 2

MANUFACTURER AND MODELS	DIAGONAL SIZE (INCHES)	DISPLAY LINES	CAPACITY CHARACTERS	CHARACTER MATRIX (DOTS)	RESOLUTION (PIXELS)	BANDWIDTH (MHZ)	HORIZONTAL REFRESH RATE (KHZ)	NUMBER OF COLORS	COMPATIBLE WITH: APPLE II?	COMPATIBLE WITH: IBM-PC?	COST
Amdek Color IV	13	24	96	5 × 7	720 × 420	16	15.75	8	Yes	Yes	$ 995
Electrohome Limited ECM 1301	13	25	80	N/A	720 × 256	25	Variable (15.75–24.6)	*	No	Yes	$1495
IBM (Systems Products Division) Color Display	12.5	25	80	8 × 8	640 × 200	14	17.75	16	No	Yes	$ 680
NEC Home Electronics (Personal Computer Division) JC1216	12	25	80	8 × 8	690 × 230	10	15.75	8	Yes	Yes	$ 695
Princeton Graphic Systems HX-12	12	25	80	8 × 8	690 × 240	15	15.75	16	Yes	Yes	$ 695
SR-12	12	25	80	8 × 16	690 × 480	25	31.75	16	Yes	Yes	$ 799
Quadram Corp. Quadchrome	12	25	80	8 × 8	690 × 480	15.0	15.75	16	No	Yes	$ 695
Sakata U.S.A. Corporation SC300	13	25	80	5 × 7	720 × 240	18	N/A	8	Yes	Yes	$ 899
SC200	13	25	80	5 × 7	640 × 240	15.0	15.75	16	Yes	Yes	$ 649
Sanyo Electric 7500	13	25	80	5 × 7	480 × 240	7	15.75	16	Yes	Yes	$ 725
Zenith Electronics Corp. (Zenith Data Systems Division) ZVM135	13	25	80	8 × 9	640 × 240	20	15.75	16	Yes	Yes	$ 599

*Only limited by the controller card.

video displays are usually limited to 40 characters per line. Some newer monochrome and RGB monitors produce more lines, more characters per line, or both. One currently available plasma display presents up to 69 lines of 160 characters per line.

Character Matrix
A dot matrix is used to make up each character in the display. The more dots in the matrix, the more legible the characters usually appear. Most current monitors use a 57 dot matrix, but 77, 79, 88, 816, 914, and 1119 are available.

Pitch
This is the distance between dots on the screen on a color monitor. The closer the dots, the crisper the display. Standard television uses a .67 mm dot pitch, while a high-resolution monitor can have a pitch as low as .31 mm (the IBM Color Display pitch is .43 mm).

Resolution
This refers to the addressable display elements (also called picture elements or simply "pixels") on the screen. These are located on an imaginary grid of coordinate lines, and resolution is therefore given in a horizontal-by-vertical format. High resolution is usually considered anything over 600 pixels horizontal. However, resolution as high as 1024 1024 pixels is now available. Monochrome monitors do not have individual display elements; monochrome resolution is listed in terms of potential display elements.

Bandwidth
Resolution is affected by the bandwidth of the signal, which is a measure of the amount of information the signal can carry. The broader the bandwidth, the more information can be carried. A monitor should be able to handle the bandwidth of the signal generated by the microcomputer to which it is interfaced. Most TV sets are limited to a 5 mHz bandwidth, while a good RGB monitor usually has a bandwidth between 10 and 25 mHz. Mismatching of the monitor and computer-generated signal can produce distortion, flickering, and a host of other problems.

Color
Monochrome monitors produce a single color, while color monitors for RGB display 8 to 16 colors, with a few specialized monitors providing more. For monochrome monitors, white and green are the most popular colors; amber is a close third in America and the most popular in Europe.

Sound
The Atari and Commodore computers generate audio output. Some monitors, most notably Amdek Color I-Plus and Zenith ZVM 135, now have built-in speakers and amplifiers to accept these audio outputs. In general, however, computer manufacturers have not opted to provide any audio output facilities beyond the computer's own speaker.

VENDORS AND COMPANIES MENTIONED

Amdek
2201 Lively Boulevard
Elk Grove Village, IL 60007
312/364-1180

Apple Computer Inc.
20525 Mariani Avenue
Cupertino, CA 95014
800/538-9696

Comrex International Inc.
3701 Skypark Drive, Suite 120
Torrance, CA 90505
213/373-0280

Dynax
5698 Bandini Boulevard
Bell, CA 90201
213/727-1227

Electrohome Limited
809 Wellington Street North
Kitchener, Ontario N264J6
Canada
519/744-7111

Hercules Computer Technology
2550 Ninth Street
Berkeley, CA 94710
415/540-6000

Hitachi America
401 West Artesia Boulevard
Compton, CA 90220
213/537-8383

IBM Systems Products Division
P.O. Box 1328
Boca Raton, FL 33432
800/447-4700

Leading Edge Products, Inc.
225 Turnpike Street
Canton, MA 02021
617/828-8150

Micro Display Systems, Inc.
P.O. Box 455
Hastings, MN 55033
612/437-2233

NEC Home Electronics
Personal Computer Division
1401 Estes Avenue
Elk Grove Village, IL 60007
312/228-5900

Panasonic Industrial Co.
One Panasonic Way
Secaucus, NJ 07094
800/222-0584

Princeton Graphic Systems
170 Wall Street
Princeton, NJ 08540
609/683-1660

Quadram Corp.
4355 International Boulevard
Norcross, GA 30093
404/923-6666

Sakata U.S.A. Corporation
651 Bonnie Lane
Elk Grove Village, IL 60007
312/593-3211

Sanyo Electric
1200 W. Artesia
Compton, CA 90220
213/537-5830

Sony Corporation of America
Sony Drive
Park Ridge, NJ 07656
201/930-1000

USI Computer Products
150 North Hill Drive
Brisbane, CA 94005
415/468-4900

Zenith Electronics Corp.
Zenith Data Systems Division
1000 Milwaukee Avenue
Glenview, IL 60025
312/391-8860

Glare Shields

With color monitors, glare can be a major problem. It is usually less of a problem with monochromes. Some monitors use a mesh across the screen to reduce the glare, but the mesh makes it difficult to clean the screen. Some of the newer monitors use an antiglare mask behind the face shield. We suggest you look at the monitor in a well-lit room and be sure that the amount of glare is acceptable.

Refresh Rate

This refers to the number of times per second the electron guns scan the horizontal display lines to refresh the phosphor's glow. The faster the rate, the less likely there is to be a flicker on the screen. The horizontal refresh rate is usually expressed in kiloHertz. RGB monitors generally tend to have the highest refresh rates.

Ergonomics

The amount of effort required to use a monitor receives more attention from European monitor designers than from those in the United States, although U.S. manufacturers are also turning to ergonomic design. If you or a staff member expect to sit in front of the monitor for long periods of time, some features to consider are these:

TILT/SWIVEL

The ability to swivel the monitor from side to side or tilt it forward or backward to maximize comfort and minimize glare can be a definite asset.

DISPLAY CONTROLS

The ability to control the brightness, contrast, and color on the screen can be important, especially as the level of ambient light in the room changes. Some monitors, like the Princeton, have few controls, while a Zenith will provide many controls on its display. Having the controls on the front rather than the back of the monitor can be helpful.

SCREEN SIZE

Given identical formats, the larger the screen, the larger and more legible the characters.

CHARACTER SIZE

The more display elements contained in the cell that is used to make up the character, the more clearly defined the character will be. Character clarity is best on a monochrome display with a monochrome board.

REVERSE VIDEO

Studies have shown that a user's pupils dilate and contract each time they move back and forth from black characters on a white paper to light characters on a dark screen. Some vendors of word processing systems have emphasized in their advertising that all-white screens with black letters have less potential for eyestrain. While the significance of this factor in the overall strain at the work place has not yet been determined, most CRT monitors will produce reverse video (also called *inverse* video).

VENDORS

Many microcomputer manufacturers (such as IBM, Apple, NEC, Sanyo, Hitachi, Zenith, Texas Instruments, DEC) provide monitors with an assured level of quality and compatibility with their computers. Do not consider price a measure of quality, however. In a recent issue of *Consumer Reports* [2], some of the cheapest monitors performed as well as or better than the more expensive ones.

Amdek is a major supplier of third-party stand-alone microcomputer monitors. It offers monochrome, composite, and high-resolution RGB color monitors, and has sold over 300,000 since 1981. Its monitors are primarily targeted at IBM-PC and Apple microcomputers.

NEC is the American marketing arm of Nippon Electric Company in Tokyo. It is the second largest third-party microcomputer monitor manufacturer, and likewise targets its monitors at the IBM-PC and the Apple, as well as the NEC microcomputer.

Princeton Graphics was founded in 1981 by C. T. Wu, and has become important in the third-party monitor market. In 1983, it merged with Intelligent Systems Corporation. The firm concentrates primarily on the IBM-PC and IBM-compatible high-resolution RGB monitors. The Princeton Graphics HX-12 and the newer SR-12 outperform IBM's own PC color display, and do so at a comparable price.

Quadram Corp was founded in 1981, and, like Princeton Graphics, has been acquired by Intelligent Systems Corporation. Its products are targeted for the IBM-PC and Apple microcomputers.

Sakata U.S.A. Corporation is the American subsidiary of an established Japanese printing-supplies manufacturer. It produces one monochrome and two RGB monitors that are compatible with the IBM-PC and Apple.

Sanyo produces a wide variety of electronics equipment. It began to sell microcomputer monitors actively in 1981, and now has an extensive dealer network. All its monitors are IBM- and Apple-II-compatible.

Sony is a very large Japanese electronics manufacturer. It produces a wide variety of very high quality monitors.

Zenith Data System Corporation was organized in 1979 when Zenith Radio Corporation acquired the Heath Company. It produces a wide cross section of monitors, all of which have received superior reviews.

SELECTING A MONITOR

TV Monitors

This is often the lowest-cost option if one can generally use an existing home television. For a recreational computer where games rather than word processing or spreadsheets are the major interest, this is an acceptable plan, though it does represent a compromise in visual quality. Some TV sets now have "computer inputs" and can deliver quality comparable to composite video monitors. A few even provide RGB color generation.

Monochrome Monitors

Most users of microcomputers will want a monochrome monitor. Monochrome is the best choice for text-oriented work, charts, and single-color graphics. The price is right—monochrome monitors that produce 80 characters per line with good resolution are available for under $100 (see Table 1). Color monitors, which are more expensive, usually produce less crisp lettering, and lower-resolution graphics.

Most monochrome monitors are interchangeable among a large variety of computers, but require the IBM's *color* monitor board. Only IBM's monochrome monitor (and a few others) require IBM's monochrome monitor board. The IBM monochrome monitor is a specially designed but expensive mate for the IBM-PC. We recommend buying the color monitor board and one of the third-party monochrome monitors. This option is much cheaper than the proprietary IBM monochrome approach, and gives you the option of switching to color later on without having to buy a new monitor controller board. However, if the majority of your work is word processing and you are satisfied with monochrome graphics, a Hercules board is highly recommended. In all cases, make sure the board and monitor are compatible.

Composite Color Monitors

These display devices are superior to the RF TV monitor, but inferior to the more costly RGB monitors. They are usually limited to 40 characters per line; and their color quality and resolution make them a poor choice for text-oriented work, although quite satisfactory for games and low-resolution software. Examples of the more popular composite color monitors are Amdek Color I plus (260300 pixels, $399), Hitachi CM 1481 (260300 pixels, $380), NEC JC-1410 (800400 pixels, $998), NEC JC-1215 (250 pixels horizontal, $399), Panasonic SR A101 (250240 pixels, $330), Sakata 100 (280300 pixels, $329), and USI C1400 (260300 pixels, $399). We think that the price of composite video is somewhat high, considering its limitations.

RGB Monitors

Because they use three separate input signals, each with a broader bandwidth, RGB monitors produce the best color output. If quality is your primary goal, an RGB monitor is the best choice. The price has been dropping dramatically over the past year, and excellent RGB monitors are now available from $600–$1000 (see Table 2).

Combination Monitors

A number of manufacturers produce monitors with both composite and RGB capabilities. This can be particularly useful if you want to have high-quality computer output and interactive video on the same screen; and some of the prices are quite attractive. Examples of these monitors include: Panasonic DTD 1300D (450240 pixels, $500), Sanyo DMC 7500 (480240 pixels, $725), Sony ZUM 131 (390240 pixels, $379), Sony KX 1901A (320200 pixels, $850), and Zenith ZVM 135 (640240 pixels, $599).

Color Graphics Boards

A color monitor frequently requires a color expansion board. This board, as well as the software being utilized, can limit your ultimate color range and resolution. For example, the IBM color display board allows only four colors at one time under medium resolution (320200 pixels), while several other vendors offer boards that display up to sixteen colors at that resolution. Be sure that your monitor and color board are compatible, and that you are purchasing a monitor with a resolution and color range which match those of your microcomputer.

Note that we have cited list prices in this report. Like most peripheral equipment, monitors can often be bought at heavily discounted prices. Shopping around can save you up to 30 percent. □

REFERENCES

1. Zuckerman MM. Innovative display technologies: why a flat panel when you can have a CRT? Compcon 1984 (Spring): 397–404 (IEEE 884 CH2017-2, IEEE Service Center Piscataway NJ).

2. How to choose a monitor. Consumer Reports 1983; 48:537–9.

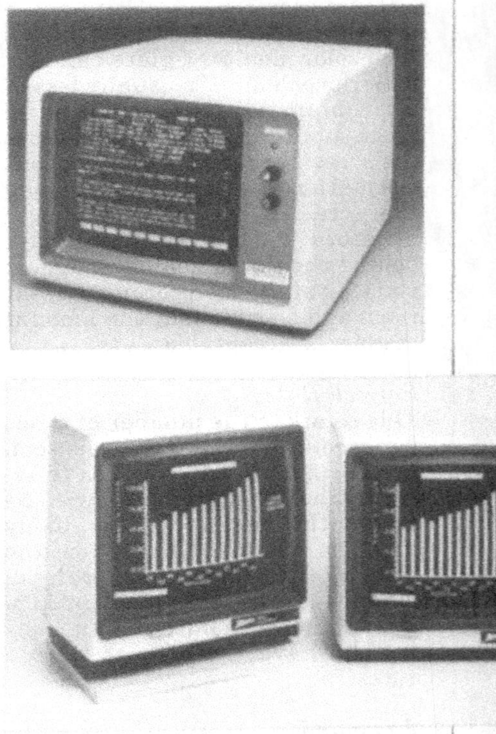

Although a color screen is useful for certain applications, business graphics can also take advantage of the shading effects that are possible on a good monochrome monitor, such as the MAX-12 from Princeton Graphic Systems (top) or the Zenith models ZDM 122 and ZDM 123 (bottom).

PRESENTATION GRAPHICS: AN INTRODUCTION AND REVIEW OF FOUR SYSTEMS

TULL T. GLAZENER AND
CLEMENT J. McDONALD, M.D.

Anyone who presents numeric data visually for a scientific paper or conference knows how hard it can be to obtain good graphics. Even if you are fortunate enough to have a medical illustrations department in your institution, it still takes your time to sketch and label the axes, and secretarial or technician time to plot the points. Then you wait. Three weeks is not rare at our institution. If you find an error, or want a different look, you wait again. The service can be expensive, and provides no opportunity for experimentation. Doing it yourself does not solve the problem. Just imagine asking an employee to throw away the finished product and try again with the X and Y axes reversed after it has taken five hours and ten restarts to get the current product. If you have ever faced these problems in presenting your data in graphic form, you should know about presentation graphics programs.

Graphics programs eliminate manual plotting and let you experiment with alternatives. You can switch from a bar graph to a line graph, reverse the axes, experiment with different scales and colors, change the text labels, and then look at the final result on the screen—all in a few minutes. With the right equipment, you can produce a paper copy suitable for publication in the most particular journal, or a set of color slides to carry to your conference. Presentation graphics programs are modestly priced ($200–$500) and are available for most 16-bit computers and the more popular 8-bit computers.

To test the usefulness of the following programs for medical graphics, we selected graphs presented in recent issues of medical journals and attempted to re-cre-

TULL T. GLAZENER
Tull Glazener is a programmer/analyst with the Regenstrief Institute, a health care research organization in Indianapolis. He has been working with a variety of mini and micro computers over the past six years, primarily for development of an automated clinical laboratory system. A frustrated artist at heart, Tull holds in high esteem anything which can draw straight lines and smooth curves effortlessly.

ate them using the graphics programs. With the exception of Figure 9, the examples presented in this report are all products of these attempts.

The programs classified under the general rubric of presentation graphics have one goal: to let you translate empiric data easily into one of a few standard graphic forms. They usually let you produce scattergrams, bar graphs, line graphs, and pie charts. These are not general-purpose graphics programs. They do not let you create arbitrary figures or three-dimensional shapes, or process images. (Future issues will review programs that perform some of these functions.)

BAR GRAPHS, PIE CHARTS, LINE GRAPHS, AND SCATTERGRAMS

There are four kinds of figures you can create with presentation graphics programs. The first is the bar graph—a series of bars whose lengths represent the value of each single variable. The histogram is the most familiar example (Fig. 1). Bar graphs come in several types. One is the comparison chart which usually shows bars in a series of clusters. Each cluster compares measurements from one or more groups of individuals. The measurements that apply to each group are distinguished by different colors or patterns of fill (Fig. 2). Another variant is the segmented bar graph. In this case, a single bar may be divided into more than one segment identifying the contribution of a number of factors to a total value. Related segments in a series of bars are identified by the same fill pattern or color. Whereas most bar graphs are vertical, the horizontal bar graph is a possible variant. Finally, there are double-sided bar graphs—two bar graphs sharing a common base (Fig. 3). Graphics programs vary in the looks of the bars they display. Most present the bar as a flat stripe, but a few show them in three-dimensional perspective.

All graphics programs also create pie charts. Their purpose is to show the relative contribution of components to the whole. This format is used more frequently in business (to show how each subsidiary contributed to company profits, for example) than in medical applications. But much clinical data could be described by pie charts: the contribution of each specialty to a clinic's total patient load, for example, or the age breakdown of patients in a clinical trial. Adjacent "slices" of the pie are filled with different colors or patterns to distinguish them. Most graphics programs permit you to emphasize any particular pie slice further by moving it away from the rest of the pie—a technique called "exploding" (Fig. 4).

The contribution of each component in a pie chart is reported as a percent. Some packages require that your data be entered as percentages. Others permit you to en-

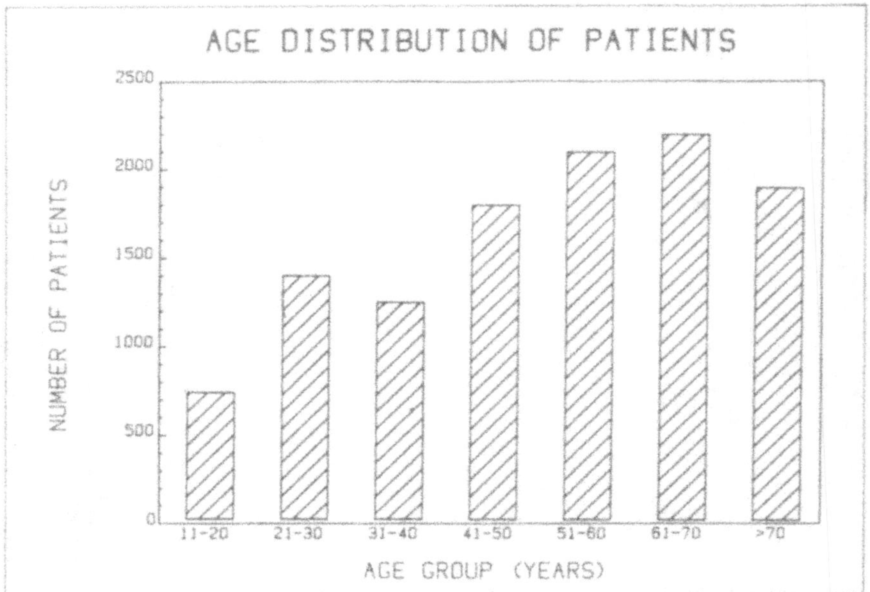

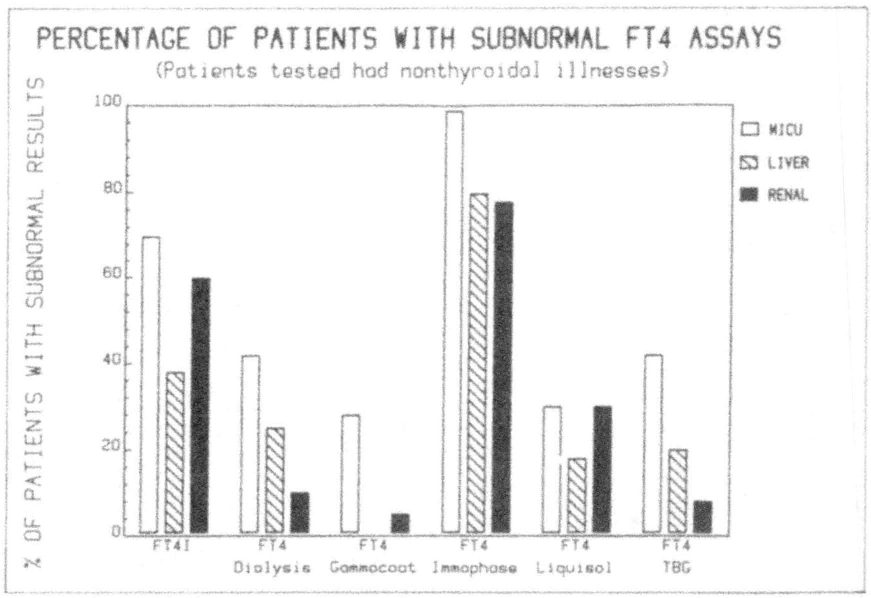

Figure 1. Histogram by GIRAPH.

Figure 2. Clustered bar graph by GIRAPH. Reproduced from *Annals of Internal Medicine,* 1983; 99:310.

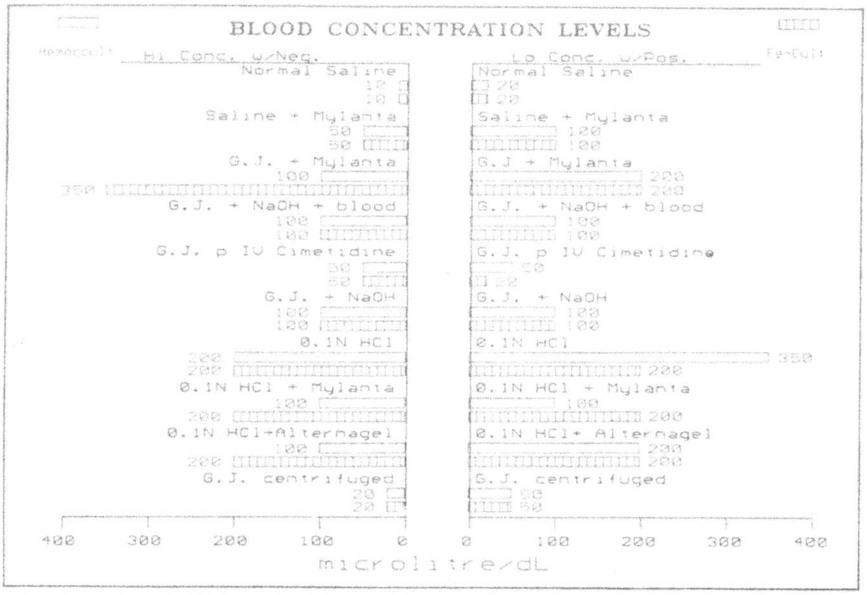

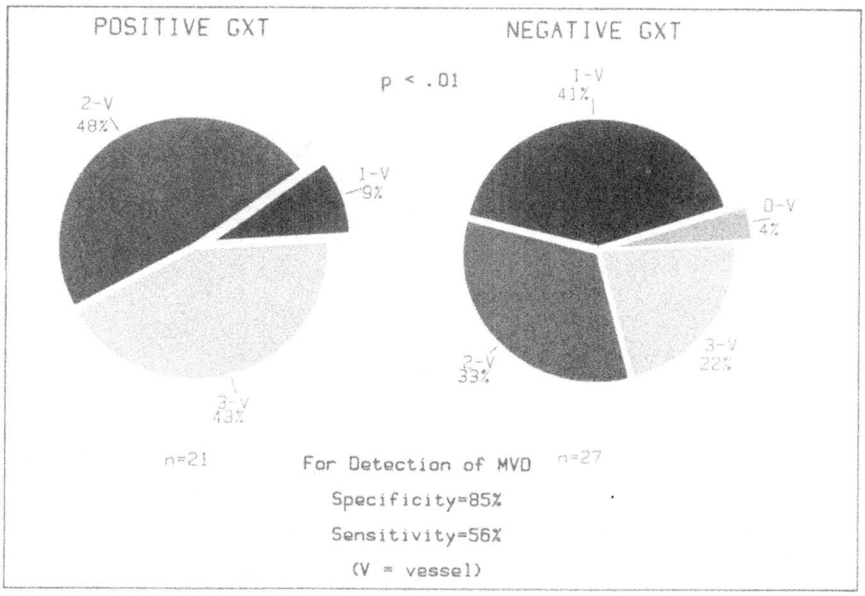

Figure 3. Doubled-sided bar graph by BGS. Reproduced from *Annals of Internal Medicine*, 1981; 94:775.

Figure 4. Pie charts by GIRAPH. Reproduced from *Annals of Internal Medicine*, 1981; 94:729.

ter raw data and they compute the percentage—a more convenient approach. One of the packages permits rotation of the pie chart after it has been created so that any one of the pie segments is on the horizontal.

Line graphs display the relationship of one variable to another. A line graph is created by plotting a series of points and connecting them by lines. Most graphics programs presume that the points are measured at regular intervals on the horizontal axis. They ask for the interval and then accept only the vertical axis values for each point. Consequently, if your data were observed at irregular intervals, you must usually use the scatter plot option to graph them.

All the programs permit choice of the character, e.g., a □ or an * that identifies the observed point on the graph, and the color and pattern of the line that connects them. Usually the choice is among solid lines, dashed lines, dot-dash lines, and so on (Fig. 5). One program lets you use two vertical axes—one on the right and one on the left—each with its own units and scaling (Fig. 6).

The most general data display is the scatter plot which displays a series of paired observations as points on the graph. In contrast to line graphs, which usually represent data having a natural order because they are observed over time, the points displayed in a scatter plot may have no natural ordering. In addition, more than one point may have the same value as the horizontal axis. Thus, it does not make as much sense to draw connecting lines (though most of the packages will connect them). Often, however, you would like to observe the trend line through these points. Some of the packages will compute the correlation between the points and plot the regression line that best "fits" the points (Fig. 7). Others go further and let you fit exponential, quadratic, or sinusoidal equations to the data and then plot this fitted curve on top of the scattergram.

ENTERING THE DATA

The computer cannot graph what it does not know, so obviously you must enter the relevant raw data into the computer. All graphics programs have tools for reading data previously recorded on electronic media, but each has its own standard input format. If your data resides in a database management system or word processor, it is up to you to recast that data in the form the graphics program can read. Now if your data is in a spreadsheet program, the process *may* be easier. Spreadsheet programs have a command for translating their data into a standard exchange format. Unfortunately, the exchange format varies with the spreadsheet program. Most graphics programs read the exchange format of one or more spreadsheet programs. If your graphics program and spreadsheet program use the same exchange format, transfer of data is simply a matter of executing a few commands. When they do not, you will have to print your spreadsheet into a text file, and then, using an editor, reformat it to suit the input format of your graphics program. Obviously, if you already have a favorite spreadsheet program, be sure to buy a graphics program that communicates with it. In many cases, the issue of data transfer is moot, since some users normally wish to represent only a few summary statistics—means or percentages, not raw data—and these can be easily entered through the keyboard.

Be aware that you may have to enter the data differently depending upon the kind of graph you are trying to produce. The graphics program usually employs the same entry sequence for bar and line graphs, but different ones for scatter plots and pie charts. Often, you cannot switch from a bar graph format to a scatter plot without reentering the data.

MISCELLANEOUS FEATURES

So far we have talked about drawing the graph itself. What about identifying the axes and writing legends? All of the graphics packages let you title the figure, label the horizontal and vertical axes, and print legends; but they differ in the kinds of lettering and the amount of text they permit in titles and legends. Some programs allow for text anywhere on the graph (a feature needed to create example graphs 4, 5, and 7), let you define the units and scales of each axis, and provide a choice of whether to include axis tick marks. Others permit change in the size and position of the graph on the plotter so that you can put a number of related graphs in a single figure.

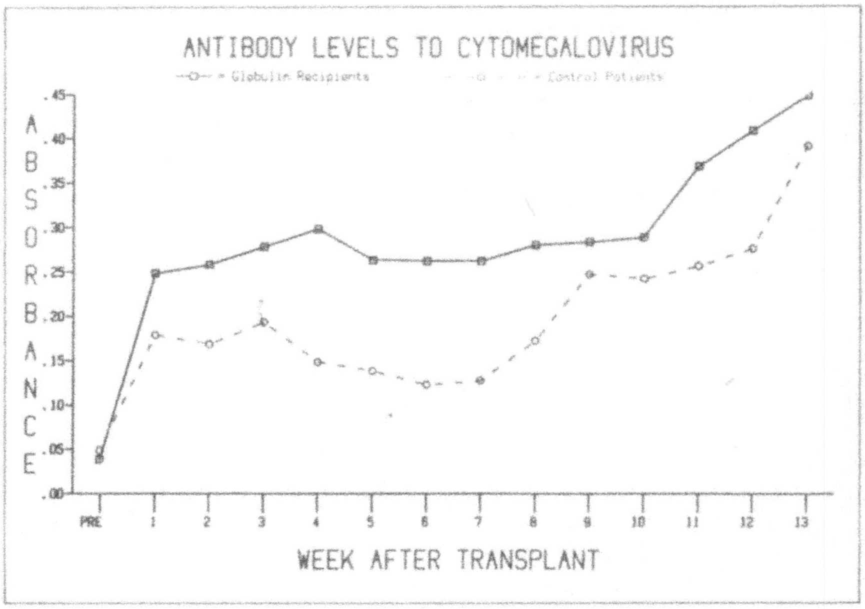

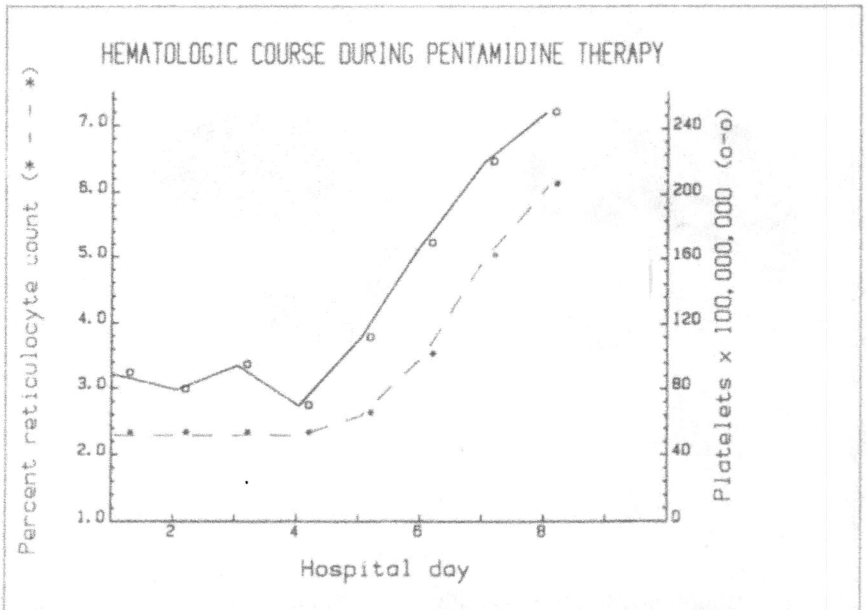

Figure 5. Line graph by BPS. Reproduced from *Annals of Internal Medicine*, 1983; 98:443.

Figure 6. Double-axis line graph by GIRAPH. Reproduced from *Annals of Internal Medicine*, 1981; 94:327.

If two or more line graphs are presented on one coordinate system (e.g., the cumulative rate of myocardial infarctions in a study group compared with the same data for the control group), each of the plotted curves needs to be identified. The same is true for many kinds of bar graphs. They are usually identified in a legend by reproducing a portion of each line or bar (using the same color and pattern that appears in the graph) and labeling it with explanatory text. Some systems permit you to locate the legend wherever you choose—a needed flexibility.

Once you have created a graph, all of the packages permit you to save on disk at least part of the work you have done. They all will save the graphic figure itself, along with its axes and legends, but some of them discard information about the position of the graph on the page, and the position of free text on the graph. This is a great nuisance if you plan to revise and reuse your graphs.

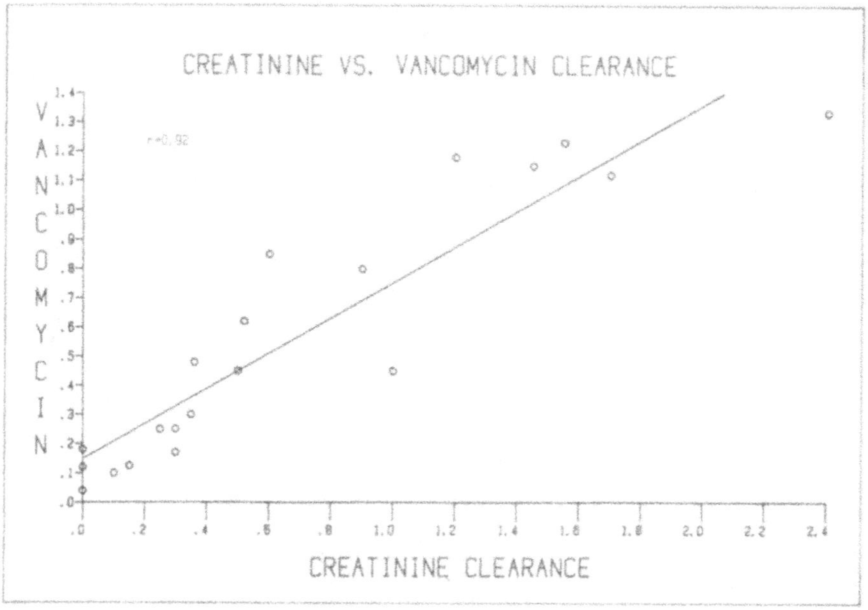

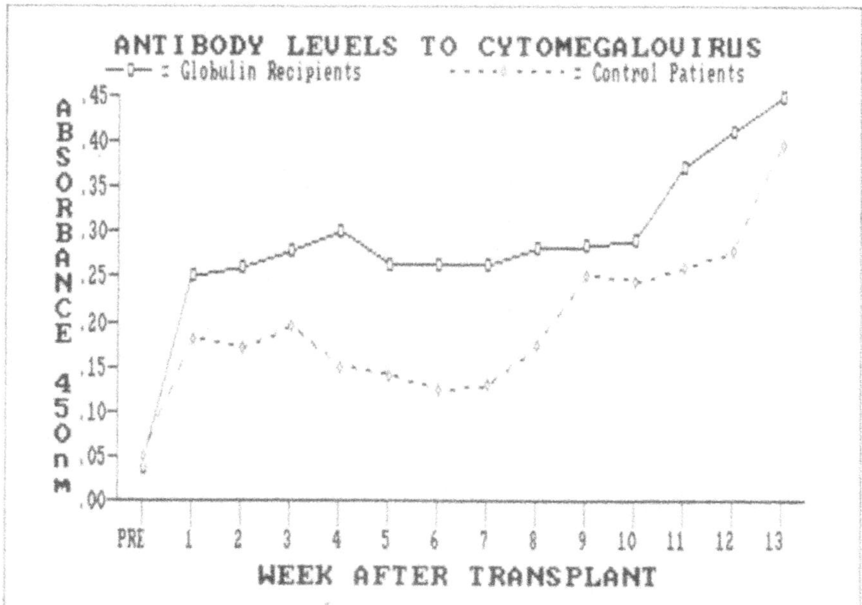

Figure 7. Scatter plot with linear regression by BPS. Reproduced from *Annals of Internal Medicine*, 1981; 94:344.

Figure 8. Line graph on a matrix printer by BPS. Compare with the identical graph done on a plotter (Figure 5).

For most conferences, you need two kinds of slides: slides for data presented in graph form, and slides for ideas presented as text. Two of the programs let you create pure text as well as graphic figures. Both give options of size, colors, and fonts of text. These systems let you produce overhead transparencies or hard copies of your slides at one pass, if you have the right equipment.

With two of the programs, you can skip slide production altogether, using an option called the "slide show." Under this option, the computer retrieves and displays the graphics you have created in a prescribed order. You press a single key to move to the next display. With this facility, you can present your material at your computer to small groups. If your conference room has the appropriate video monitors, you could even use this mechanism to present your data to a large group. We predict that such electronic displays of data will replace slide projectors in the future.

CREATING HARD COPIES OF YOUR GRAPHS

All of the programs will display your graphs on your video monitor. In the early stage of graph development, the video monitor is used exclusively. When they are installed, some of the programs assume you are using a color monitor; two of them provide no easy way of telling the computer otherwise. As a result, the characters of the graph-generating program are illegible on a monochrome monitor. We chose a monochrome monitor because of its lower price and crisper characters; and we think the vendors should make it easier to use monochrome video screens with their products.

In general, the major reason for producing a graphics display of your data is to show it to someone else, either at a conference or in a paper. Consequently, you need a hard copy device in addition to your video monitor. The choices come down to three: matrix printer, plotter, or video camera. If you own a computer that runs version 2.0 of MS/DOS (IBM-PC), you can obtain hard copy of any graphics displayed on your screen simply by pressing the "print screen" key. Four-color matrix printers, comparable in price to black ribbon printers, are now available. We tested one of these but found its print quality to be below that of the monochrome matrix printers. Moreover, it insisted on shrinking the size of the color figure to half the full page size. Nonetheless, it is an inexpensive way to obtain color hard copy and would find useful applications.

In general, the quality of graphic output from dot matrix printers does not match that of a professional graphics department. Both the text characters and the curves have a stair-step appearance (Fig. 8). These would be quite suitable for internal reports and local conferences. But for a professional look, you need one of the more expensive options.

Graphics plotters are the second major option for a hard copy output. Capable machines are priced in the \$1,000–\$2,000 range. The curves they draw are smooth, not sawtooth, and the text characters are fully formed. With the proper care, you can produce professional quality graphics and output suitable for publication with these devices. Buy a machine with a liquid ink, not a ballpoint pen. The latter is cheaper but the results are less professional. To get good copy, you must invest in the right kind of paper. Paper that is too cheap will bleed or smear. These machines can also draw on acetate, and thus you can obtain transparencies suitable for overhead projectors. You should also give some thought to the size of the pen point you use in the plotter. The finest pens produce pretty graphics, but the figure will be too thin for viewing if projected.

We used a Hewlett-Packard 7470 two-pen plotter in our test, and were quite happy with the results. You can obtain more than two colors with this plotter by changing pens during the plotting. A large variety of plotters are now available (see Table 1). Some control the use of as many as eight pens in a single pass.

Finally, the last hard copy devices to consider are photographic devices. These cover a broad range in complexity and quality. The simplest devices are cameras that bolt onto the front of your video screen (\$150–\$300, both Kodak and Polaroid instant CRT screen cameras). Moderately priced devices, from \$1500 to \$2500, take the electronic signal from the computer and use analog techniques to generate the picture. With these you can obtain brilliant colors, including those that are not available on your computer's palette. But the image you will get is what you see on your video screen. If your screen is low-resolution, the pixels will give the same stair-step appearance to the graphics that you see in the matrix printer output. The most expensive devices (\$5,000–\$8,000) use digital techniques to generate the picture. These improve the resolution of the screen image and can produce exquisite quality photographs up to 8" × 10" in size. With electronic cameras you can obtain your own slides in minutes if you use instant 35 mm film. The more expensive versions would be good investments for any graphics department. The analog cameras will produce excellent photos only if you have a very high resolution video monitor. For most clinicians who wish to make hard-copy graphics, we think the moderately priced plotters are the best choice.

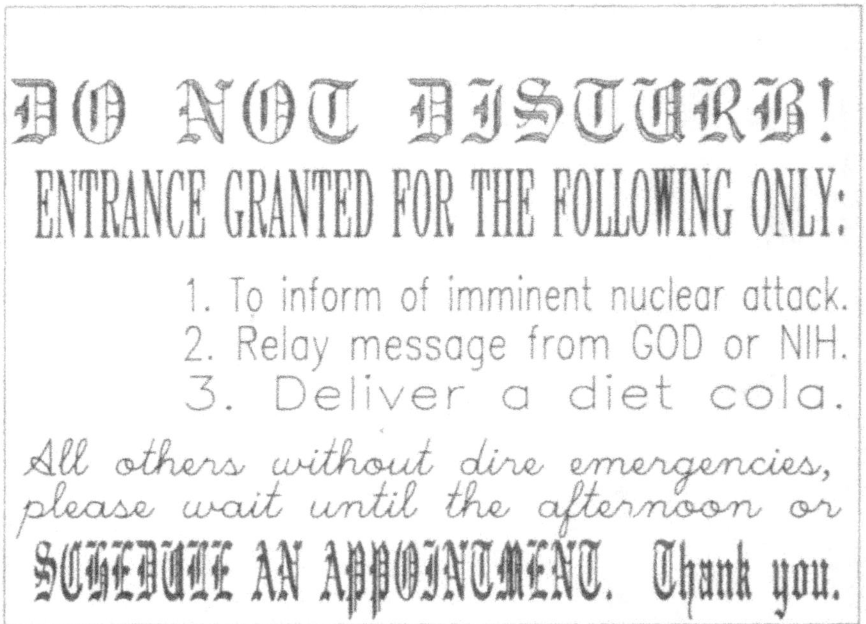

Figure 9. Free text chart by BGS.

FOUR GRAPHICS PROGRAMS IN DETAIL

We reviewed four popular packages: GIRAPH (Data Display Business Graphics Systems), BGS (Peachtree Software, Inc.), The Draftsman (Star Ware Corporation), and BPS Business Graphics (Business Professional Software, Inc.). We tested the programs on an IBM-XT with 128K of memory, standard ten megabyte disk drive. The computer included IBM's color graphics monitor adaptor board. We did not have a color monitor, which caused us some problems in installing a few of the packages. Hard copy was obtained from the Epson FX-80 dot matrix printer, a Transtar 315 color printer, and a Hewlett-Packard 7470 graphics plotter.

GIRAPH

The GIRAPH package is easy to install. Through a series of menu selections, it asks you what kind of monitor you have, the type of plotter you are using, and the color pens in each pen stall. GIRAPH "remembers" this information, so you do not have to reenter it each time you start the program.

GIRAPH's formal documentation is sparse. However, the program operation was simple enough that this was not a problem to us (and an improved manual is now being prepared). In the current version, 2 one-page "addendum" accompanies the documentation. It contains several important corrections and explanations which would take considerable time to discover on your own.

GIRAPH is fast—the fastest of any of the packages we tested (the average delay between screens was less than 1.5 seconds). It permits the freest use of text on graphs, and is the only one of the tested programs that lets you print characters parallel to the vertical axis the way they appear on most published graphs. Two other unique features are the abil-

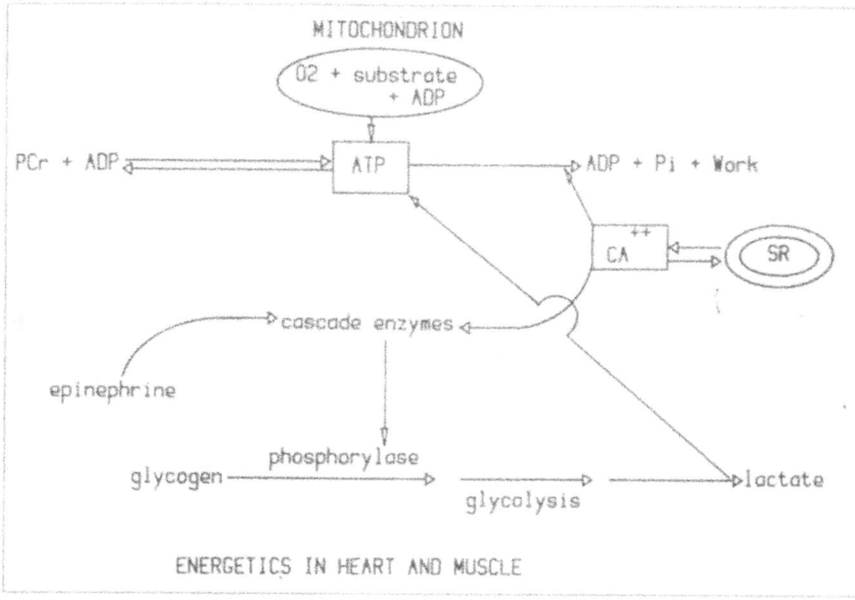

Figure 10. Free form diagram by DRAFTSMEN. Reproduced from *Annals of Internal Medicine*, 1983; 98:518.

ity to print two vertical axes on the same graph (see Fig. 6) and the step-line option.

It also permits you to create text charts. You can write up to 16 lines with 48 characters apiece and choose the size and color of the lettering. The program will automatically center or left- or right-justify each line. This option was easy to use, and the available font sizes were just right for slides (most typewriter print is too fine). GIRAPH also has a "slideshow" option. You can store up to 50 images in your electronic "carousel" and play them back on your monitor in predefined order. Two function keys control the use of three foreground and eight background colors, which can be used anytime you are using the display screen.

GIRAPH does not provide any curve fitting. Thus, if you want to print regression lines on your scattergrams, you must choose another package. The program had a few minor problems. You cannot save the position of annotating text on the graph when you save the graph. You must reposition it each time you create the graph. There were a few minor problems with editing data to be displayed, and we were bothered by the lack of pattern in the legend that identifies the curves or bars in the graph. (The legend includes only the color of the line or bar.) The vendor tells us these problems are being corrected.

BGS

BGS comes configured for a specific computer (e.g., an IBM-PC or a Zenith Z100 computer) and the HP 7470 plotter—the one we used. It also assumes you have a color monitor. Unfortunately, the complete procedures for telling the computer otherwise only appear on the screen, and if you have a monochrome monitor, you cannot read the screen. We were able to find the system configuration file (SYSTEM.CNF), and used a text editor to change the first line from Y to N. Thereafter, all was well.

The documentation was extensive but not always helpful. The pace of the tutorial section was agonizingly slow. Type A personalities should avoid it. The Quick Start section also missed its mark. It is great for demonstrating sample graphs but does little to tell you how to create your own. The reference section of the manual is excellent; it is complete and well indexed.

BGS is menu-driven and generally easy to use; however, we are bothered by some of the menu option choices. The numeric codes for fill patterns, line types, and line markers had no mnemonic content, and we had to consult the reference manual frequently to identify the options. BGS was slow to switch between menu options. The worst delay was an unpardonable 20 or 30 seconds when waiting to initiate the edit option.

BGS has a number of special features. It is the only package that offered double-sided bar graphs (Fig. 3). You can create three-dimensional bars, and specify top or bottom and left or right perspective. Like GIRAPH, BGS offers free text charts; however, you must position each line of text at an *x/y* coordinate. This is more flexible but more difficult to use than GIRAPH. BGS provides the most extensive choice in the kinds, sizes, and shapes of text. It gives you the choice of seven different font types, including triple density, cursive, and gothic, the last of which is great for making signs (see Fig. 9 for a sign used to reduce traffic into an office). You may specify not only the character size and font, but also the spacing, slant, angle, justification, direction, and placement coordinates for each line of text. BGS will also compute and plot the linear regression line through scatter plots.

We did not encounter any program errors when running BGS, but were frustrated by the limitation on lengths of label and title in the graphic options. BGS also restricts you to one set of data points to be graphed on a scatter plot, and provides no options for drawing a connecting line between these points. Its technique for specifying the use of multiple pens on a plotter is awkward. Since the line graph option under BGS requires evenly spaced points, it provides no way to draw a line graph when observtions are made at varying intervals.

DRAFTSMAN

On installation, Draftsman, like BGS, assumes you have a color monitor. The good news is that Draftsman provides a procedure you can follow for changing the configuration even though you cannot read the screen. The bad news is that the configuration data is not saved anywhere, so you

TABLE 1 MODERATELY PRICED PLOTTERS

PRODUCT & COMPANY	TYPE	# COLORS ON LINE	MAX. AREA	MEDIA	PRICE
BAUSCH & LOMB HIPLOT DMP-40 Bausch & Lomb Houston Instrument Division 8500 Cameron Rd. Austin, TX 78735 512-835-0900	drum	1	9.25″ × 15″	paper, vellum, acetate, mylar	$995
CALCOMP MODEL 84 Calcomp Inc. 2411 W. La Palma Anaheim, CA 92803 714-821-2541	flat-bed	8	11.3″ × 8″	paper, film	$1995
ENTER COMPUTER SWEET-P Enter Computer Inc. Suite D 6867 Nancy Ridge Dr. San Diego, CA 92121 619-450-0601	roller-drive flat-bed	1	8″ × 12.1″	paper, acetate	$795
H.P. 7470A Hewlett-Packard Co. Inquiries Mgr. 1820 Embaradero Palo Alto, CA 94303 800-547-3400	roller-drive flat-bed	2	7.5″ × 10.7″	paper, film	$1095
IBM XY/750 IBM Instruments Inc. Orchard Park P.O. Box 3325 Danbury, CT 06810 800-243-7054	flat-bed	8	11″ × 17″	paper, vellum, acetate	$1995
NUMONICS 5412 Numonics Corp. 418 Pierce St. Landsdale, PA 19446 215-362-2766	friction-rollers	1	10″ × 36″	paper	$1295
RADIO SHACK MULTI-PEN Radio Shack 300 One Tandy Ctr Fort Worth, TX 76102 (call local Radio Shack Computer Store)	flat-bed	6	7″ × 9.25″	paper, film	$1995
YOKOGAWA PL100 Yokogawa Corp. of America 2 Dart Rd. Shenandoah, GA 30265	cut-sheet feed	4	10″ × 15″	paper, film	$1150

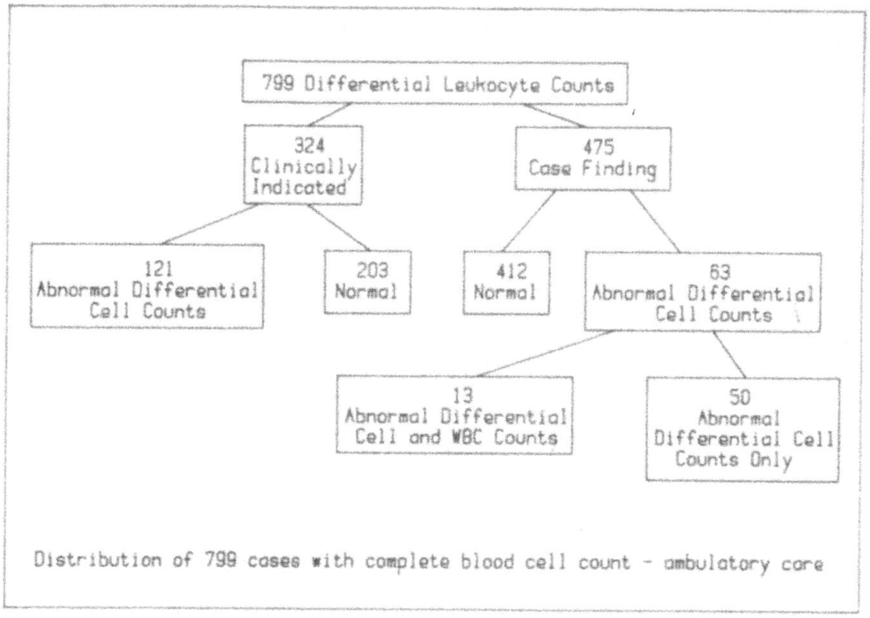

Figure 11. Free form diagram by DRAFTSMEN. Reproduced from *Journal of the American Medical Association*, 1983; 249:634.

must repeat this process each time you initiate the program. The Draftsman has the most convenient documentation of any of the programs we tested. The entire manual is provided on-line. When you have problems at any point in the program, pressing the F1 function key causes the appropriate page in the manual to be automatically displayed on the screen. You can then scroll forwards or backwards a page at a time, or jump to any other specified page.

Like the above two programs, Draftsman is menu-oriented and easy to use. It has one feature that none of the others provide: it permits you to create figures. You use single letter commands to draw dots, lines, circles, and squares, or to connect them by lines or arrows. You can create these figures in any size, and position them anywhere on the screen (Fig. 10). In addition, you can stretch or shrink circles and squares along one axis to create ovals, ellipses, and rectangles. You can overlay these shapes and graphic text on the same screen. The system also permits "freehand" drawing. You use the four arrow keys in an Etch-a-Sketch–like fashion to generate an arbitrary curve. Each press of an arrow key extends the line an additional pixel in the direction specified by the key. With the use of auto-repeat keys, it is easy to draw vertical and horizontal lines with this technique; but drawing curves or diagonals requires considerable dexterity. For arcs, it is much easier to create an oval and then erase all but the segment that one needs. Draftsman also includes a slideshow option, with the added feature of an "automated timer" between slides.

For routine presentation graphics, however, Draftsman is missing a number of important features. It does not permit the drawing of incremental tick marks or grid lines, and you cannot override the automatic scaling. It prints the label for the vertical axis horizontally near the top of the graph rather than parallel to the vertical axis. This is not the way professional graphs are drawn, and wastes much space that could be better used by the graph itself. Draftsman provides only two shading patterns for the screen, and only one of these works on the HP 7470 plotter. It provides line graphs, bar charts, and pie charts; it does not permit graphing scatter plots.

BPS

BPS is the only graphics package that is not menu-oriented. To create a graph in BPS, you write a set of individual commands—something like writing a simple program. Since it has more than 100 command variations, this approach may seem intimidating. In actual practice, only a handful of commands with appropriate modifiers are needed to produce most graphs, and these are easy to learn.

BPS is different in another way from the other programs. As we understand it, it is written in UCSD Pascal and it runs in the standard UCSD operating system under MS/DOS. This makes the program compatible with many different computers, thus explaining its widespread availability. The disadvantage—and this is slight—is that the files it creates are not directly accessible to other programs in MS/DOS.

A special command file, START-UP, is automatically executed each time the program is started. This file tells your program about your computer: the type of monitor you have, the default disk drive, etc. This is a nice feature.

The tutorial provides clear examples to help you get started. This part of the manual is supplemented by an excellent section with over 70 sample graphs and a discussion of the commands needed to generate them. Many of these examples are included on an on-line demonstration diskette. BPS does provide a help facility, but the messages are often too short to be helpful. The reference section of the manual is excellent, providing full details of the command syntax; moreover, it discusses the hardware interfaces and the software options available in a comprehensive manner. BPS supports more than 80 printers and plotters, a larger variety than any of the other programs.

This program offers the largest range of facilities of any we tested. Its curve-fitting commands are especially powerful. You can fit your data to lines, logarithms, exponentials, and parabolas. The program not only provides the parameters for the best-fitting curve, it displays the equation, curve, actual fitting curve, and a statistical measure of how close the fit is. It provides for curve

TABLE 2 GRAPHICS PROGRAMS' FEATURES

BAR GRAPHS	GIRAPH	BGS	DRAFTSMAN	BPS
#groups/observations	14/60	5/12 or 2/32	5/32	unlimited
clustered	yes	yes	yes	yes
stacked	yes	yes	yes	no
horizontal	no	yes	no	yes
3-dimensional	yes	yes	no	no
#fill patterns	24	9	4	6
double-sided	no	yes	no	no
LINE GRAPHS	**GIRAPH**	**BGS**	**DRAFTSMAN**	**BPS**
#groups/#observations	14/60	5/12 or 2/32	5/32	unlimited
line markers	any keyboard character	any keyboard character or 6 special symbols	5 special. symbols	8 special symbols
line types	3	5	1	5
plot points only	no	yes	yes	yes
step-line	yes	no	no	no
area graphs	yes	yes	no	yes
thick lines	yes	no	no	no
PIE CHARTS	**GIRAPH**	**BGS**	**DRAFTSMAN**	**BPS**
# slices	14	12	12	unlimited
explode slices	yes	yes	yes	no
leave out missing slices	no	no	no	yes
rotate	yes	no	no	no
data as degrees	yes	no	no	yes
SCATTER PLOTS	**GIRAPH**	**BGS**	**DRAFTSMAN**	**BPS**
#data sets/points	7/60	1/183	---------	unlimited
choose point symbol	no	yes	---------	yes
connect points	yes	no	---------	yes
fit line	no	linear regression	---------	constant, line parabola, log exponential, sine

smoothing of your raw data using weighted or unweighted averages. You can also tell the program to generate new points, to take your own data and predict the extrapolated or future trends of a curve fit.

The commands provide features very similar to those of a programming language. You can manipulate data arithmetically (e.g., divide one variable by another) or normalize your data within the language. This is a facility very much like mainframe statistical packages. The only limitation is that arithmetic operations must be performed one step at a time.

The system lets you save a series of commands you used to produce a complex graph, storing them in a named disk file. These commands can be executed automatically by invoking the name. You can then edit existing files to create new graphs or link together a whole series of files to create a slideshow, although there will be a considerable delay between images while the graphs are redrawn.

BPS requires somewhat more learning investment than the menu-oriented programs, but the command language provides greater flexibility and power. Using it does not require programming experience, although a scientific background would certainly help. BPS runs reasonably fast; however, you experience a long delay between the time you initially load the program and the time you can enter your first command—nearly one minute in our system. There are also noticeable delays between various segments of the graph production. Graphs seem to run faster if the commands are obtained from a previously created command file than when typed into the keyboard.

Our major criticism of BPS relates to the production of hard copy output: it does not let you specify the location of the graph on the output device. This means you cannot put multiple graphs on a single page. Nor can you control the size of the graph. In addition, it is difficult to produce fill and shading patterns permitted on the HP 7470 plotter. BPS is the only package that lets you access data directly from any text file (such as those created by spreadsheet programs, word processors, or database management systems), but it

FORMAT OPTIONS	GIRAPH	BGS	DRAFTSMAN	BPS
grid lines	yes	no	no	yes
tic marks	yes	yes	no	no
override scaling	yes	limited	no	no
draw a frame	yes	yes	yes	no
2 vertical axes	yes	no	no	no
maximum label size	60	15–20	20	60
free text	yes (plotter only)	no	yes	yes
control size & placement	yes	yes	yes	no
control plotter pen speed	yes	yes	no	yes
SPECIAL FEATURES	**GIRAPH**	**BGS**	**DRAFTSMAN**	**BPS**
text charts	yes	yes	limited	limited
slide show	yes	no	yes	limited
data manipulation	no	no	no	yes
transparency formatting	yes	no	no	no
DATA ENTRY	**GIRAPH**	**BGS**	**DRAFTSMAN**	**BPS**
keyboard editor	yes	yes	yes	yes
text files	fixed format	fixed format	fixed format	any format
spread sheet programs	MULTIPLAN, VISI-CALC	PEACH CALC	- - - - - - - - -	MULTIPLAN direct, any other via text files
INSTALLATION	**GIRAPH**	**BGS**	**DRAFTSMAN**	**BPS**
	Easy	Assumes color monitor/HP7470	System type, not stored	Special command file
DOCUMENTATION	**GIRAPH**	**BGS**	**DRAFTSMAN**	**BPS**
	Sparse	Mixed	Most convenient	Excellent
SPEED	**GIRAPH**	**BGS**	**DRAFTSMAN**	**BPS**
	Fast	Slow	Moderate	Reasonably fast/ some delays
PRICE	**GIRAPH**	**BGS**	**DRAFTSMAN**	**BPS**
	$190	$295	$200	$350

requires that you build a form description telling BPS exactly where each of the data values is located in the file. This is a powerful feature, but we found it very difficult to use. It took nearly as long to master this one technique as to become familiar with all the other commands on the system.

For creating command files, BPS provides a full screen character editor; for entering data, it provides only an old-fashioned line editor. The line editor is functional, but far more difficult to use than modern screen editors.

SUMMARY AND CONCLUSIONS

Table 2 summarizes the features available in each of the four packages we reviewed. Each package has its own strengths and weaknesses, and your choice will depend upon your requirements. For routine graph making, we prefer GIRAPH. It is the easiest to learn (it took less than five minutes to teach two physician colleagues to use it); it is the fastest and easiest to use, and most often produced exactly the graph we wanted.

If your work requires curve fitting, then BPS is by far the best. It has the greatest number of features, can be used with the greatest number of printers and plotters, and is available on more types of computers than any of the others. BGS has the most extensive lettering capabilities, and would be preferred by those who need special lettering on their graphs or signs. It also should be considered by those who want an integrated system, since it is part of an overall package that includes a spreadsheet program, a word processor, a list processor, and other word managing programs.

The Draftsman is also easy to learn, but is missing a number of features required for the usual presentation graphics. However, it is the only one that lets you draw on your graphs—ideal for showing relationships among structural, chemical, or logical components (see Figs. 10 and 11).

These are only a few of the many graphics programs available across a variety of microcomputers. Many of those not tested have excellent features. There are also graphics capabilities in so-called integrated programs—those containing spreadsheets, database

PACKAGES REVIEWED

GIRAPH
Data Display
171 West 4th Street
New York, NY 10014
(212) 620-8134
Price $190

BGS
(Business Graphics System)
Peachtree Software, Inc.
3445 Peachtree Road, N.E., 8th Floor
Atlanta, GA 30326
(800) 247-3224
Price $295

The DRAFTSMAN
Starware
1511 K Street, Suite 1150
Washington, DC 20005
(202) 331-8833
Price $200

BPS Graphics
Business & Professional Software, Inc.
143 Binney Street
Cambridge, MA 02142
(800) 342-5277
Price $350 (approx.)

managers, and graphics programs—that permit shifting from one program to another without moving data.

Should you buy a separate graphics program such as one of those described here or use the graphics in one of the integrated packages? It is obviously easier to manage data in the integrated packages. However, current versions do not offer as many capabilities as the specialized graphics programs, and for presentation graphics, you generally will need one of the specialized programs. This could all change. The integrated packages are likely to enhance the graphics capability with time. On the other hand, it is also quite possible that interface standards will develop so that specialized programs will have no more difficulty in exchanging data with other programs than will programs within integrated packages. We hope the latter occurs. We are much more likely to obtain exactly the programs we need if the diversity of specialized program vendors continues, so that we can pick the best programs for our own particular purposes and yet interchange data between them. □

PUTTING DOCTORS BEHIND BARS

TULL T. GLAZENER AND CLEMENT J. McDONALD, M.D.

A few years ago, if you asked the man on the street to define "bar codes," he might have mentioned anything from the codified ethics of lawyers to the dress requirements at a drinking establishment. Today, however, more and more people understand them to be the stripes, printed black on white, that adorn supermarket products ranging from cat food to breakfast cereal.

Easily read and decoded by computers, bar codes have found a wide range of applications. They have been used to identify and track items ranging from boxcars to luggage and from groceries to marathon runners. The use of bar codes has also been proposed for identifying chickens, artifacts at archeological digs, and pilgrims traveling to Mecca. Of more relevance to physicians, bar codes have been used to identify hospital patients, blood bank samples, laboratory specimens, X-ray folders, and medical record charts.

Bar code symbols can be read either by passing a wand over them or by passing the labeled items themselves over the reader. Wanding of bar code information has two major advantages over manual keying of the same information. It is twice as fast as a high-speed typist, and ten times faster than an untrained one. It is also more accurate: one error per million characters, compared to one error per thousand characters for an experienced keypunch operator. Of course, bar code identification is only practical when the object you want to identify can be labeled with a bar code. The cost of producing the bar code label and applying it to the object must be considered when deciding whether to employ bar codes in an application. Bar code identification can most easily be justified when an item must be identified several times during its passage through the system.

Today, sophisticated wands—ranging in cost from $600 to $1000—are available for reading bar codes into microcomputers. Bar code readers designed for use with a computer terminal can be plugged into the system in such a way that the computer can't tell whether the entered characters were typed in or wanded by a bar code reader. Some microcomputer bar code readers provide similar capabilities. More importantly, with appropriate programming, most microcomputer matrix printers can print bar codes. Thus, if you are using a microcomputer for billing, you could print labels showing the patients' names and chart numbers in standard text and in bar code symbols, apply these labels to the corresponding charts, and then identify the patients to the computer by wanding the bar codes on their chart labels when you enter billing transactions during their visits. No changes whatsoever would be re-

TULL T. GLAZENER
Tull Glazener is a programmer/analyst with the Regenstrief Institute, a health care research organization in Indianapolis. He has been working with a variety of mini- and microcomputers over the past seven years, primarily for the development of an automated clinical laboratory system.

CLEMENT J. McDONALD, M.D.
Dr. McDonald is a professor at the Indiana University School of Medicine, Director of Computer Science Research at the Regenstrief Institute for Health Care in Indianapolis, and a practicing internist. Over the past ten years he has developed computerized pharmacy, clinical laboratory, and medical records systems at Wishard Memorial Hospital in Indianapolis. His major research interest is the effect of computerized reminders on physicians' behavior. His book, Action-Oriented Decisions in Ambulatory Medicine *(Chicago: Year Book Medical Publishers, 1981) summarizes this work.*

quired in your billing program.

Most hospital medical record and radiology computer systems identify charts and X-ray folders, respectively, with bar codes. Likewise, many clinical laboratories use bar codes to identify specimens as they pass through the various processing stations of the lab.

Two proposed uses of bar codes could be of special value to computer hobbyists and scientists. The first is to print the computer programs that appear in computer magazines in bar code symbols, as well as in text, so that interested readers could enter whole programs by wanding the magazine pages instead of typing them in. Some editors have proposed that the author, title, and sources of journal articles be printed in bar code symbols, as well as standard text, so that physicians and scientists could maintain their reprint collections on computer by wanding in these bar codes. Finally, it has been suggested that laboratory and X-ray results be reported to physicians' office computers in bar code, as well as in text. Such bar-coded laboratory reports could be entered into an office practice computer by wand much more efficiently than by keyboard entry.

You may conceive of other uses of bar code readers for your practice. So we thought it would be worth explaining how bar codes work, and presenting a program for printing them. The program illustrates an approach that could be applied to any printer with graphic capabilities.

CHAR.	PATTERN	BARS	SPACES	CHAR.	PATTERN	BARS	SPACES
1		10001	0100	M		11000	0001
2		01001	0100	N		00101	0001
3		11000	0100	O		10100	0001
4		00101	0100	P		01100	0001
5		10100	0100	Q		00011	0001
6		01100	0100	R		10010	0001
7		00011	0100	S		01010	0001
8		10010	0100	T		00110	0001
9		01010	0100	U		10001	1000
0		00110	0100	V		01001	1000
A		10001	0010	W		11000	1000
B		01001	0010	X		00101	1000
C		11000	0010	Y		10100	1000
D		00101	0010	Z		01100	1000
E		10100	0010	-		00011	1000
F		01100	0010	.		10010	1000
G		00011	0010	SPACE		01010	1000
H		10010	0010	*		00110	1000
I		01010	0010	$		00000	1110
J		00110	0010	/		00000	1101
K		10001	0001	+		00000	1011
L		01001	0001	%		00000	0111

Figure 1. ***Code 39*** **Code Configuration. The ★ symbol denotes a unique start/stop character which must be the first and last character of every bar code symbol. Reprinted from David Allais,** ***Bar Code Symbology: Some Observations on Theory and Practice*** **(1982), courtesy of INTERMEC Corporation.**

ABC

1234-5

123-45-6789

SM4592-3

Figure 2. Bar code printout produced by the bar code printing program.

HOW DO BAR CODES WORK?

There are many different standard systems for defining bar codes. Each system is referred to as a "symbology." Perhaps the most familiar symbology is that of the UPC (Universal Product Code) symbol which was adopted by the supermarket industry in 1973 [see "The Search for National Standards for Medical Data Exchange," *M.D. COMPUTING* 1(1):3]. Other popular symbologies include: EAN (European Article Numbering); *Code 39*, also known as *3 of 9 Code*; CODABAR; and *Interleaved 2 of 5*. While the names of these codes suggest exotic and complex methods of encoding information, in each case the actual means by which the wand reader interprets the code is fairly simple.

All of the information in a set of bar code symbols is carried by the relative widths of the bars and intervening spaces. The height of the bars contains no information. Information is represented in bar codes as binary patterns (or bits) in all bar code symbologies. The only differences among the various symbologies concern the rules for encoding this binary information. For example, in one symbology a narrow bar printed on the label might represent a *0*, and a wide bar a *1*, while in another symbology, the width of the white spaces may also encode a binary digit (*0* or *1*). Alphanumeric characters are represented by sequences of binary codes, just as in internal computer memory. For example, in *Code 39*, the letter *A* is represented by bars and spaces that read *100001001*.

All bar code readers illuminate the code with a bright light. Black bars absorb the light, and white bars reflect it back to the scanner. The scanner transforms the patterns of light and dark into time-varying electrical impulses (analog signals) that correspond to the relative widths of the white and black spaces on the bar code. The decoder in the reader transforms these patterns into standard ASCII codes that are transmitted to the computer just as if they were being typed in at the keyboard. When a bar code reader is connected to a computer, data can be entered from either the computer's keyboard or the bar code reader, and the computer will make no distinction.

Symbologies vary in the number of digits or characters that can be included in the bar-coded "message." Some symbologies are of fixed length; that is, every bar code label contains the same number of characters. Others permit a variable number of characters to be included in the message; these symbologies add special codes to indicate the beginning and the end of the bar-coded message. Some symbologies always include extra digits or characters to verify the accuracy of the bar code reading. Such systems have extremely low error rates.

Code symbologies vary in the kinds of information that can be transmitted. Some permit only numeric data, while others permit alpha and numeric data in their messages.

HOW CAN I IMPLEMENT A BAR CODE APPLICATION?

Entering information by wanding a bar code—instead of by typing in the same information—generally requires no programming, since most bar code readers transmit the data so that the computer behaves as if the data *had* been typed in. Before you can use bar codes, you have to generate labels to identify your items in a bar code form. This can be done with most popular matrix printers that have graphics capabilities.

Because of *Code 39*'s internal structure, it is one of the most reliable bar code symbologies, and the most tolerant of minor irregularities in the printing of the black bars. For this reason, *Code 39* bar codes, printed by a matrix printer, can be accurately read. Another advantage of *Code 39* is the fact that it has been adopted by the Department of Defense as a standard, thus assuring its long and widespread use.

Code 39 bar codes can be printed in densities ranging from one to ten ASCII characters per inch. Ten characters per inch is as dense as standard typewriter print. However, the ratio of wide to narrow widths must be between 2:1 and 3:1, and the intercharacter gap should be the same width as the narrow bands. (See Figure 1 for the complete set of symbols.)

On the following two pages, we present a program for generating *Code 39* symbols on the Epson FX or MX series of dot matrix printers. The program converts any string of input text to the corresponding bar code pattern, and prints both the bar codes and the original text. (The accompanying notes give a step-by-step explanation of the program.)

The program is written in MicroSoft BASIC for the IBM-PC, and will run on any MS/DOS computer. Samples of the program's output are shown as Figure 2. We tested the bar codes printed by this program with an Intermec model #9300 bar code wand reader.

Also, you may recall that the grocery checkout clerk sometimes has to pass a package over the reader more than once to get a confirming beep. The same is true if a wand reader is used: the reader does not always see the pattern correctly at the first pass. When the reader does "understand" the code, it signals its acceptance by a beep. The first-read success rate for the bar codes printed by our program was approximately 98%. This success rate depends upon the person who does the wanding, as well as the quality of the printed bar codes. We have found that

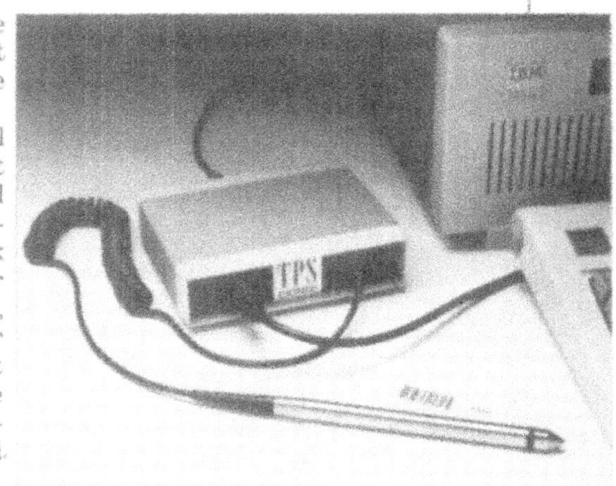

the wand scanning motion should be done with a gentle, even wrist swing to achieve the highest first-read rate. With a little practice, this comes naturally. □

VENDORS OF BAR CODE READERS

Bar/Code Inc.
1251 Exchange Drive
Richardson, TX 75081
1-800-527-4719

CAERE Corporation
100 Cooper Court
Los Gatos, CA 95030
408/395-7000

Computer Identics Corporation
5 Shawmut Road
Canton, MA 02021
617/821-0830

Identicon
(A Division of Vertex Industries)
23 Carol Street
P.O. Box 1123
Clifton, NJ 07014
201/473-6900

Intermec Corporation
4405 Russel Road
P.O. Box C-N
Lynwood, WA 98036-0694
206/743-7036

Skan-a-Matic Corporation
Route 5W, P.O. Box S
Elbridge, NY 13060
315/689-3961

Symbol Technologies, Inc.
1101 Lakeland Avenue
Bohemia, NY 11716
516/563-2400

TPS Electronics
4047 Transport Shelf
Palo Alto, CA 94303
415/856-6833

BARCODE PRINTING PROGRAM

PROGRAM NOTES

Lines 50–72: These data statements define the *Code 39* character set. Each character consists of five bars separated by four spaces. "1" indicates a wide bar or space; "0" indicates narrow.

Lines 100–170: This section reads in the character set. As each character is read in, a flag is set (line 150) to indicate that the character is a valid *Code 39* character. The loop from 155 to 158 reads the five bar elements; the loop from 160 to 165 inserts space elements.

Lines 180, 185: These are the bit patterns for printing a vertical space [CHR$(0)] and a vertical line [CHR$(254)] on the Epson printer. There are eight pins on the Epson print head; they can be controlled individually. These are numbered in powers of 2 from bottom to top (1, 2, 4, etc.). 254 is the sum of the powers of 2 for the bottom seven pins. (We are using seven-pin graphics, instead of using all eight pins, so that the program will work on eight-bit computers as well.)

Line 190: If you are running under MS/DOS, the default width of the line printer is 80 characters, and MS/DOS will try to insert <CR><LF> for you unless you change the width. When in graphics mode, MS/DOS counts each column of dots as one character.

Lines 200–210: We are using a 2½:1 ratio of wide elements to narrow. This is accomplished by printing a symbol five dots across for wide elements and two dots for narrow. (Changing these constants will change the density of your symbol; just be sure to maintain a relative ratio of between 2:1 and 3:1.)

Line 220: The total number of dots that we will print for each character is computed here. Three wide elements, six narrow elements, and an intercharacter gap make up each character.

Lines 230–240: To print a row of graphics on the Epson printer, you must first enter a "graphics mode," and then tell the printer the number of columns you wish to print at one time. The *N2* argument reserves "bunches" of 256 dots, while the *N1* argument contains the number of single dots left over after the groups of 256 have been print-

```
1     'This program accepts a string of characters from the
2     'user (keyboard) and translates it into CODE39 bar code
3     'for the EPSON (or IBM) family of printers.
5     'Note that the printer must be connected to the first parallel
6     '(synchronous) port, or otherwise designated as "LPT1:"
30    DIM      CODE(256,9), OUT.PUT$(1), B$(50)
45    '-------------------------------------------------------------
46    ' The following data statements describe the CODE 39 character set.
47    ' After each character, a group of 5 numbers describes the BAR pattern,
48    ' while the next group of 4 numbers describes the SPACE pattern.
49    ' A "1" indicates a wide bar or space, while a "0" indicates narrow.
50    DATA     " ",0,1,0,1,0,  1,0,0,0,  "-",0,0,0,1,1,  1,0,0,0
51    DATA     "$",0,0,0,0,0,  1,1,1,0,  ".",1,0,0,1,0,  1,0,0,0
52    DATA     "*",0,0,1,1,0,  1,0,0,0,  "%",0,0,0,0,0, 0,1,1,1
53    DATA     "+",0,0,0,0,0,1,0,1,1,   "/",0,0,0,0,0,  1,1,0,1
54    DATA     "0",0,0,1,1,0,  0,1,0,0,  "1",1,0,0,0,1,  0,1,0,0
55    DATA     "2",0,1,0,0,1,  0,1,0,0,  "3",1,1,0,0,0,  0,1,0,0
56    DATA     "4",0,0,1,0,1,  0,1,0,0,  "5",1,0,1,0,0,  0,1,0,0
57    DATA     "6",0,1,1,0,0,  0,1,0,0,  "7",0,0,0,1,1,  0,1,0,0
58    DATA     "8",1,0,0,1,0,  0,1,0,0,  "9",0,1,0,1,0,  0,1,0,0
60    DATA     "A",1,0,0,0,1,  0,0,1,0,  "B",0,1,0,0,1,  0,0,1,0
61    DATA     "C",1,1,0,0,0,  0,0,1,0,  "D",0,0,1,0,1,  0,0,1,0
62    DATA     "E",1,0,1,0,0,  0,0,1,0,  "F",0,1,1,0,0,  0,0,1,0
63    DATA     "G",0,0,0,1,1,  0,0,1,0,  "H",1,0,0,1,0,  0,0,1,0
64    DATA     "I",0,1,0,1,0,  0,0,1,0,  "J",0,0,1,1,0,  0,0,1,0
65    DATA     "K",1,0,0,0,1,  0,0,0,1,  "L",0,1,0,0,1,  0,0,0,1
66    DATA     "M",1,1,0,0,0,  0,0,0,1,  "N",0,0,1,0,1,  0,0,0,1
67    DATA     "O",1,0,1,0,0,  0,0,0,1,  "P",0,1,1,0,0,  0,0,0,1
68    DATA     "Q",0,0,0,1,1,  0,0,0,1,  "R",1,0,0,1,0,  0,0,0,1
69    DATA     "S",0,1,0,1,0,  0,0,0,1,  "T",0,0,1,1,0,  0,0,0,1
70    DATA     "U",1,0,0,0,1,  1,0,0,0,  "V",0,1,0,0,1,  1,0,0,0
71    DATA     "W",1,1,0,0,0,  1,0,0,0,  "X",0,0,1,0,1,  1,0,0,0
72    DATA     "Y",1,0,1,0,0,  1,0,0,0,  "Z",0,1,1,0,0,  1,0,0,0
99    '-----------------------------------------------------
100   '*************** INITIALIZATIONS ******************
120   FOR I = 1 TO 44                       ' 44 characters in Code39 set
130          READ C$                         ' read character
140          C = ASC(C$)                    ' convert to ASCII numeric equivalent
150          CODE(C,0) = -1                 ' set flag saying this character found
155          FOR J = 1 TO 5                 ' loop thru bar element pattern
156                 READ CODE(C,J*2-1)  ' read bar element pattern
158          NEXT J
160          FOR J = 1 TO 4                  ' loop thru space element patterns
162                 READ CODE(C,J*2) ' read space element pattern
165          NEXT J
170   NEXT I
180   OUT.PUT$(0) = CHR$(0)              'Bit pattern to print a space
185   OUT.PUT$(1) = CHR$(254)            'Bit pattern to print bar (top 7 dots)
190   WIDTH "LPT1:", 255                 ' prevents DOS from inserting <CR><LF>
200   NWIDE = 5                                'Print 5 dots for wide bar/space
210   NNARROW = 2                              'Print 2 dots for narrow bar/space
220   NTOTAL = (3*NWIDE) + (6*NNARROW) + 2 'Total # dots for each character
221                                            ' (There are 3 wide elements and
222                                            ' 6 narrow elements in each
223                                            ' Code39 character, plus 2 spaces
224                                            ' between each character.)
230   N2 = NTOTAL/256                         'Compute # of groups of 256 dots.
240   N1 = NTOTAL MOD 256                     'Get # dots remaining after line 230
```

```
250   GS$ = CHR$(27) + "L" + CHR$(N1) + CHR$(N2)
251                                         'This string kicks the EPSON into
252                                         'low-speed double-density graphics
253                                         'mode, allocating the correct number
254                                         'of graphics characters for one
255                                         'Code39 bar code character.
260   PRINT CHR$(27)"1"                     'Set EPSON for 7-dot line spacing
999   '---------------------------------------------------------------
1000  '---------------- C O N T R O L   R O U T I N E ---------------
1010  INPUT "String to convert";S$      'Get string to convert to Code39 format
1015  IF S$ = "X" THEN GOTO 31000        ' "X" means to stop the program
1020  S$ = "*" + S$ + "*"                'Add start/stop characters to string
1030  L = LEN(S$)                        'Get total length of string to convert
1070  FOR I = 1 TO L                       ' loop thru each character in string
1080            C$ = MID$(S$,I,1)        ' break single character out of string
1085            C = ASC(C$)                 ' Get ASCII code for this character
1090            IF CODE(C,0) = 0 THEN GOTO 1100
1091                                          ' Skip this character if not allowed
1092                                          ' in Code39 set
1095        GOSUB 2000                       ' Convert character into Code39
1100  NEXT I
1110  FOR H = 1 TO 3                         ' Loop thru string 3 times to give
1111                                          ' a height of 21 dots.
1120      FOR I = 1 TO L                     ' Loop thru characters in string.
1130          LPRINT GS$;B$(I);            ' Print Code39 string preceded by
1131                                          ' EPSON graphics control code.
1150      NEXT I
1160      LPRINT                              ' Force a <CR><LF>
1170  NEXT H
1180  LPRINT " ": LPRINT S$ : LPRINT " ": LPRINT " "
1185                                          ' Print text in human-readable form
1190  GOTO 1000                              ' Get next string to convert.
1499  '---------------------------------------------------------------
2000  ' ************** convert character to bar-code format ***************
2005  B$(I) = ""
2010  FOR E = 1 TO 9                         ' each character has 9 elements
2020          X = (E AND 1)                  ' odd #s are bars, even are spaces
2030          FOR L2 = 1 TO 3*(CODE(C,E))+2 ' 5 dots for wide, 2 for narrow
2035                  B$(I) = B$(I) + OUT.PUT$(X) ' print dot or space
2040          NEXT L2
2050  NEXT E
2060  B$(I) = B$(I) + OUT.PUT$(0) + OUT.PUT$(0) ' add space between character
2090  RETURN
2099  '---------------------------------------------------------------
31000 ' ****************** exit routine ****************************
31010 CLOSE
32767 END
```

ed. In our case, since we will be printing each character separately, we always print 29 dots across for each bar code character.

Line 250: CHR$(27) + "L" is a special escape command sequence that tells the Epson to shift into low-speed double-density graphics mode. This will give us a nice solid bar with (we would hope) smooth edges.

Line 260: This escape command tells the Epson to print each line seven dots high. Again, this is for the convenience of our friends with eight-bit computers.

Lines 1000–1015: These statements prompt the user to supply the desired string to convert into *Code 39* bar code. Our convention is to keep asking the user for another string until the user types an *X*.

Line 1020: Here we append the special start/stop character (the "*") to the beginning and ending of the string.

Line 1030: Figure out the total number of characters in the string.

Lines 1070–1100: In this loop, we look at each individual character in the string and check whether it is a valid *Code 39* character (remember, this program does not support the full ASCII character set). If it is not valid, it simply is ignored. Otherwise, we perform the subroutine at line 2000 to convert an ASCII character into its *Code 39* equivalent. (The details of this routine follow.)

Lines 1110–1170: Once the characters have been converted, we print the entire *Code 39* symbol three times on successive lines, giving each character a height of 21 dots. This height is a personal preference, and simply makes it easier for a human to wand the bar code by allowing for a greater margin of "hand wavering" error. Note that the inner loop at lines 1120–1150 prints each bar code character without a terminating line feed/carriage return sequence. (This is accomplished by the terminating semicolon.) 1160 forces a line feed/carriage return each time the entire symbol has been printed.

Line 1180: Here we print the string in human-readable form and double-space to get ready for the next symbol.

Subroutine 2000: Convert a single character to *Code 39* format.

Line 2005: Initialize *Code 39* string for this character.

Lines 2010–2050: Loop through nine elements of each character. The odd-numbered elements are bars, which are printed as vertical lines. The even-numbered elements are spaces. Line 2020 causes *X* to be set to 0 or 1, depending on whether it is an even- or odd-numbered element. We use *X* as an index to the graphics output strings initialized in lines 180–185 to print a vertical line (bar) or space.

Lines 2030–2040: *L2* is computed to be the width of the element. If the element is wide, five dots will be printed; if narrow, two dots.

Line 2060: Here we add the white space for the intercharacter gap at the end of each character.

LET YOUR COMPUTER DO THE TALKING AND THE LISTENING

WILLIAM PEARSON, Ph.D.

Today, your personal computer and your telephone make a mighty pair. You can use the two to search the scientific literature as it is stored on the giant bibliographic systems (see M.D. COMPUTING issue 0), review national financial data, or capture the stock market ticker tape (and automatically save selected data for charting stocks). You can also exchange programs with amateur computerists on a national network or connect your computer to a neighbor's to transfer files or programs or simply dial up your office computer from your home. The setup for talking to another computer requires some special equipment and understanding of how the process works. On your end, you will have to have a modem, a special cable, and usually, a communication program, all of which have to be properly "connected." The connections are not difficult, but without some knowledge of how and exactly what should be connected, the process can be frustrating. We will save you this frustration by explaining how these components work and interrelate.

William R. Pearson is an Assistant Professor of Biochemistry at the University of Virginia School of Medicine, Charlottesville. His research interests are in molecular biology and the control of gene expression in mammalian cells. He uses micro- and mainframe computers to locate patterns in DNA sequences. In addition, he has been hooking up little computers and calculators to bigger computers for the last 8 years to avoid having to learn how to type.

THE PHYSICAL CONNECTION

To talk to an outside computer, you need four things: a telephone, a modem (modulator-demodulator), a cable, and either a VDT (video display terminal) or a computer (with its own keyboard and video display screen). Most of this discussion will be devoted to computer-to-computer communication, but because some of you may want to use a terminal to talk to a remote computer, we will discuss use of the terminal as well.

CABLING

Most terminals and microcomputers transmit data through cables connected by standard 25-pin connectors. The male plug is called a

DB25/P. The female socket is called a DB25/S (see Figure 1 photograph). Most microcomputers send data in serial form; this means the information bits move through the wire one behind the other like a series of box-cars and only one wire is needed to send information in one direction. But with only one wire for data, the computer communication would have the same limits as a two-way radio: information could only be sent in one direction at a time. Most computers permit simultaneous two-way communication. In fact, even what appears to be one-way communication, i.e., from a keyboard to your computer, is usually two-way. What you type on your keyboard does not go directly to the screen; it goes to the computer and the computer "echoes" it back to the screen. The same applies to communication between a VDT (video display terminal) and a computer. What you see on the screen has traveled from the keyboard to the computer and back to your screen. The advantage is that you see what the computer picked up, allowing you to spot transmission errors. This communication mode is called duplex, and the two-way nature becomes most apparent when it stops, which occurs, for example, when you type a secret password that is not echoed back on the screen.[1]

To send and receive signals at the same time, the connecting cable must have at least two wires—one for sending and one for receiving. A third and fourth wire (a safety ground and a signal ground, respectively) are also usually needed. An EIA standard for cabling specifies exactly which pin should be used for what function in the cable. The zero and the seventh pin are used for safety and signal ground, respectively. The second and third pins are used for sending and receiving, respectively. Figure 2 shows the minimum cable needed to connect a VDT to a modem (the box that converts the computer's digital signals to telephone signals). Notice the numbers in the figure. These identify the pins. If you look carefully at the face of a connector, you can see similar numbers embossed above or below some of the pins on a male connector and in comparable positions on the back of a female connector. (If you really want to know what is connected to what at each end of the cable, you must remove the connector covers and examine the color-coded wires.) What is described in Figure 2 works for a VDT terminal. It will not succeed if you use your home computer to call up an outside computer. Why not?

Communication specialists refer to VDT printers and other such devices as data termination equipment (DTE), and they refer to computers and modems, i.e., machines that generally send information to terminals, as data communication equipment (DCE). Terminals and other kinds of DTE receive data on pin 2 and send data on pin 3. Computers and modems (DCE) do just the opposite: they send data on pin 2 and receive it on pin 3. The cable needed for connecting a computer to a host computer, either directly or via a modem, is shown in Figure 4. Note the crossover of the wires connecting pins 2 and 3. Such a cable is referred to as a null modem. The general rule is that when connecting two DCE devices or two DTE devices, cross the connections between pins 2 and 3. When connecting a DCE device with a DTE device, connect pin 2 to 2 and 3 to 3.

So far we have described the use of only 4 of the 25 pins on the standard connector. Most of the 25 pins have a purpose. Many computers, printers, and terminals require that some of these other connectors be wired, meaning more wires in the cable. The most commonly used of the 25 pins are those shown in Table 1.

The additional lines are used to signal that the device is ready to receive or transmit data or that the modem is correctly linked to the phone line. Like the send and receive lines, many of them come in pairs: request to send and clear to send; data terminal ready and data set ready. When these pairs of signals are required, they follow the same rule as the send and receive lines, i.e., if the cable connects like kinds of equipment (DCE to DCE or DTE to DTE) the wires must cross within each pair, e.g., pin 4 to 5 and 5 to 4 (see Figure 4). If the cable connects "opposites," the wires connect the same pins, e.g., pin 4 goes to 4 and 5 to 5. Some devices need these to be connected and some do not. Most of the remaining pins are used to control special features of modems and are not needed by most home applications.

Getting the right cable to connect two devices can be a problem. Depending upon the devices, you may need cables with 4, 8 or even more wires and the exact connection required will vary. To further complicate the situation, computers are sometimes configured to be DTE instead of DCE devices. Moreover, vendors do not always follow the pin assignment standards and often choose the plug type (male or female) without regard to the standards. It seems to be a rule of nature that the cable you have is never the one you need for a new piece of equipment. One solution to the cable problem is to buy a cable from your vendor that is *guaranteed* to connect the two devices you own. But vendors tend to charge exorbitant prices for cables—$30–$40 for a 5–6 foot cable is common. A cheaper solution is to use special adaptors and standard 4-wire telephone lines. The adaptors plug into the RS232 sockets on your equipment and have receptacles for the standard telephone jacks. (We know of at least one vendor, Dorlabs of Harvard, MA, that provides these adaptors.) They will work in most cases, but you have to know enough about your equipment to specify which of the eight different adaptors you need. Finally, with a soldering gun

[1]Communications modes in which data can be transmitted and received independently are known as "full duplex". The "half duplex" mode does not automatically echo characters as they are sent. In half duplex, the terminal (or the modem) sends the characters back to the screen as they are typed and the host computer receives only the characters. This method is used by some large IBM computers not well-suited to acting as each individual character is received. Unfortunately, because the display may show the correct character even though an incorrect character was received, errors in the communications circuit are not easily detected.

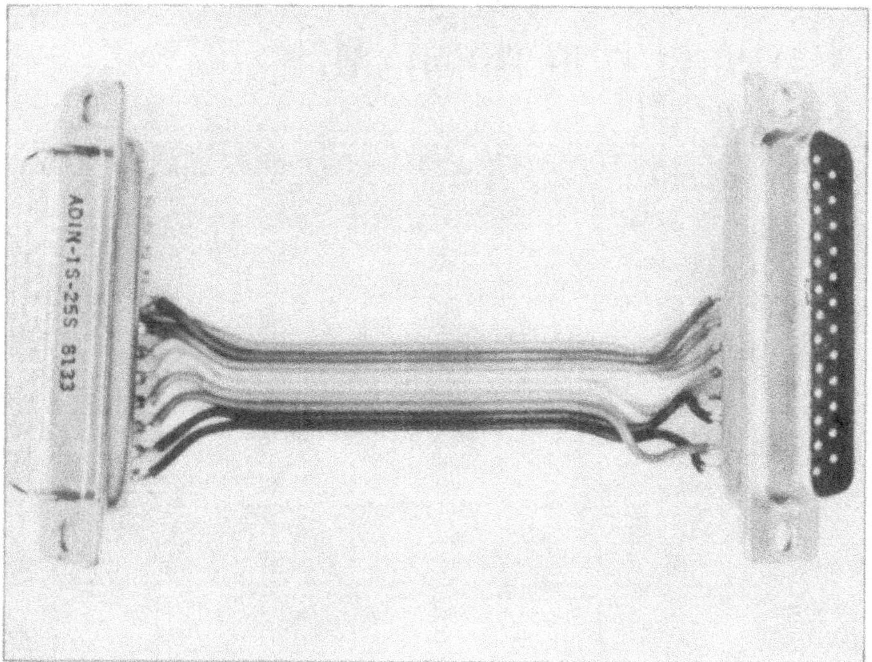

Figure 1 Photograph of two cable connectors

or crimping tool, you can wire your own cable.

COMMUNICATIONS SPEED

Computer-generated text is transmitted as ASCII (American Standard Code for Information Interchange) code. Large (but not small) IBM computers use EBCDIC as their code. ASCII is simply one way of assigning a code number to the upper and lower case letters of the alphabet, the digits 1 through 9, and punctuation marks. The full set of codes is shown in Table 2 (the ASCII table). The ASCII code includes several characters not found on standard typewriters, such as the tilde '~' and vertical bar '¦'. Ninety-five code numbers are assigned to printable characters. The remaining 33 numbers are control characters, including backspace (8), tab (9), carriage return (13), line feed (10), and delete (127). On many computer terminals these characters control such special functions as cursor movement on the screen or screen erasing.

To send the character "A", a computer sends A's ASCII code—the number 33—as a series of ones and zeros. The binary representation of "A" (33) is 100001. Since the other characters, such as "a" (65, 1000001) need a seven-place binary code, all ASCII codes are sent as groups of at least 7 ones or zeros. Thus, "A" is encoded 0100001. Since these ones and zeros flow through the connector one after the other as a series of voltage changes, the process is called *serial communications*, and the sending device is called a *serial RS232 port*[2]. The RS232 standard defines a mark (binary 1) as a voltage between −3 and −37 volts and a space (0) as a voltage between +3 and +37 volts. Thus the letter 'A' becomes a stream of positive and negative, 5-volt signals: −5, +5, +5, +5, +5, −5, +5. But this stream is not sufficient because without some timing information, the terminal or modem cannot distinguish +5, +5, +5, +5 from a single +5. Timing information is important because most ASCII-based communications are asynchronous: you press a key, wait, then press several keys in quick succession, so that the interval between the transmitted characters varies. The positive or negative pulses that result are of fixed duration.

The interval between these pulses determines the communications speed. Common speeds are 300 or 1200 bits per second (baud) for telephone communications and 9600 baud for a terminal connected directly to a computer. At 300 baud, a single one or zero (−5 or +5 volts) lasts for 3.3 msec. Since it usually requires 10 bits to send an ASCII character[3], 300 baud is equivalent to 30 characters per second. Twelve hundred baud, or 120 characters per second, is the fastest telephone communications speed possible without special modems and software. At 300 baud, text can be comfortably read as it is received. At 1200 baud, you must stop the text occasionally to read it. Generally, you will want the fastest speed you can get.

Successful communication is possible only if both systems are communicating at the same speed. Mismatched communications speeds are easy to diagnose because you will see that characters on your screen bear no relationship to the transmitted text. Often, unusual characters appear such as "~~~\\\{}}××××××."

THE TELEPHONE CONNECTION

A terminal connected directly to a computer can transmit signals with −5 and +5 volt pulses; however, communications over long distance use sound signals transmitted over telephone lines. A modem converts transmitted voltages to sound and reconverts the sound to

[2]Many printers use an alternative method called *parallel communications* which transmits all 7 bits at once, and therefore requires at least 7 wires.

[3]In addition to the 7 bits required to encode a character, 1 bit is used to signal the start of a character (start bit), another to signal the end (stop), and a third is often used for error checking (parity). Different computers require different combinations of data and parity bits. The most common configuration on large computers is 7 data bits and even or odd parity. "Even parity" means the number of ones in the 7 + 1 bits is an even number. For example, "A" (0100001) has two ones, so the parity bit would be 0, making the total number of ones an even number. Microcomputers usually expect 8 data bits, so that not only 7 bit text but also 8 bit bytes can be sent, and no parity bit.

voltages. Two types of modems are in common use: *slow speed* (up to 300 baud, Bell 103 compatible, costing between $100 and $250) and *high speed* (up to 1200 baud, Bell 212 compatible, costing between $500 and $900).

Slow speed modems modulate the computer's digital signals into pairs of "voice grade" tones: one pair uses 1270 cycles per second (Hz) for a one and 1070 for a zero; another uses 2225 Hz for a one and 2025 Hz for a zero. One frequency pair is needed for transmitting data and another for receiving data. If you listened in to a telephone sending these signals, you could hear these tones as music-like warbling. A computer terminal is connected to a modem in an "originate mode." The distant computer is then dialed. Its modem, in "answer mode," responds with a tone. In this case, the 1070/1270 pair transmits data and the 2025/2225 pair receives data. If both modems were accidentally in originate mode, both would transmit using the 1070/1270 pair and neither would hear the other. This situation is the same as having two computer terminals transmitting to one another over the same connector pin. Just as there must be DTE and DCE connectors, there must be "originate" and "answer mode" modems.

Higher communications speeds require more sophisticated technology and the high speed modems are therefore more expensive. One type, the Bell 202 compatible, is not really suitable for microcomputer communications, yet they are advertised for microcomputers. Two other types, the VADIC 3400 and the more popular Bell 212 modems, can be used with microcomputers, but they are not compatible with each other.[4] If you plan to spend lots of time using other computers over the telephone, then the higher priced high speed modem is worth it. The slower ones work well for short calls to check messages or record financial information.

[4]A Vadic 3400 modem cannot talk to a Bell 212 type, but triple modems, which use the low speed 103 protocol and both the 3400 and 212 high speed protocols, are available.

CONNECTING TERMINAL TO MODEM

Figure 2 Schematic of minimum cable for connecting terminal to modem (or any DCE with any DTE)

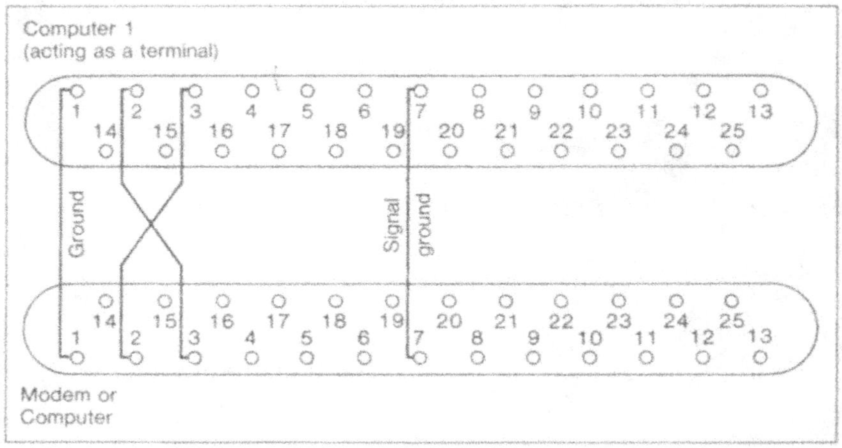

Modems are available as originate only, originate/answer and auto-answer types. Originate/answer modems can switch the tones used to send or receive data so that they can either dial up other computers or be dialed up. An auto answer modem can answer the phone.

Recently, intelligent modems such as Hayes Smartmodem™, have been introduced. These contain a microprocessor that can dial other modems or answer the telephone. With an intelligent modem, therefore, you can dial up your computer and use it from a remote location.

COMMUNICATIONS SOFTWARE

Microcomputers talk to other computers by acting like computer terminals. In addition to the normal keyboard and screen, the microcomputer masquerading as a terminal must have an additional communications connection, called a serial RS232 port, to the distant computer. These ports or interfaces are available for most popular microcomputers. If your computer does not have one, a serial RS232 printer port can often be adapted.[5] A parallel printer port cannot be used for modem communications.

Communications programs connect the microcomputer keyboard to the transmitter section of the communications port and link the receiver section to the microcomputer screen. You would find the following logic in a simple communications program:

Loop: If a key has been pressed, get the character and send it to the communications port.

If a character is ready at the communications port then get the character and send it to the screen.

Go back to loop.

A communications program constantly checks the keyboard and communications port to see if a character is ready to be sent or is ready for the screen. It does not wait for a character from either source; it checks, loops, checks, loops, etc., and it can work only as fast as the slowest output device. As a result, if the communications port was receiving data at 120 characters per second but the screen could display only 60 char-

[5]In this case you would make a null modem consisting of two DB25P male plugs connected by crossing the 2/3, 4/5, 6/20 pin pairs.

acters per second, half of the characters would be lost. For computers with separate terminals, this is usually not a problem, but for some computers with integral displays, such as the IBM-PC and the Apple, high speed transmission can be a problem. These computers use a more sophisticated programming technique, "interrupt driven" input/output, and programs for the IBM-PC can communicate up to 9600 baud.

More advanced computer communications call for your microcomputer to do more than a simple computer terminal. The most useful advanced communications function of most communications programs is the ability to record on the disk data sent to the screen. By capturing data on a disk as it is displayed on the screen, any information—literature references, lab reports, financial data—can be saved for future manipulation and reference. For example, if you access information about a new drug for hypertension, but you are overwhelmed with references to other diseases in which the drug is also indicated, you could pare down the number of references by using more specific terms, or you could save all the references and use your word processor to search the references for keywords related only to hypertension. Thus, you could save a large number of references to the drug, references which might include contraindications not yet associated with hypertension.

Recording data on the disk requires a simple modification of the basic logic of our communications program. Take the program outline shown earlier and simply add the option of sending the data to the disk and the screen.

```
Loop: If a key has been pressed, get the character and send it to the communications port.

      If a character is ready at the communications port then get the character and send it to the screen, and if recording, then send the character to the disk.

      Go back to loop.
```

CONNECTING HOME COMPUTER WITH A SERIAL DCE

Figure 3 Schematic of minimum cable for connecting home computer with a serial DCE (printer) connector (used to call remote computer) to a modem. (Same applies to other DCE to DCE or DTE to DTE connections.)

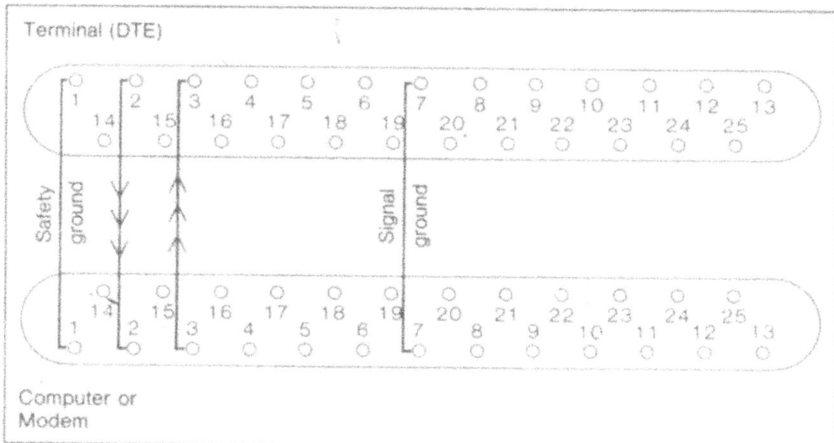

The process of sending a character to the disk, however, is slightly more complicated than sending one to the screen. Magnetic disks store information in blocks of from 128 to 1024 characters. The characters must be stored in memory until there are enough to completely fill a block. Since the disk is a mechanical device, time is required to start the disk drive, move the recording head, and actually record the data. During this time, the characters coming into the communications port may be ignored and lost. Communications programs prevent this by storing the characters in the computer's memory and writing them to the disk only when the memory is filled or the recording session is over. Storing characters directly in memory is much faster than sending them to the screen, so characters are not ignored and lost. Storing information in memory before it is sent to the disk (or to any other device, such as a printer) is called "buffering."

By using a "buffer," a communications program can store about 32,000 characters, or 500 lines of text, before actually saving the text or the disk. Simple programs are limited to saving blocks of 32,000 characters or less to prevent loss of data when text is finally sent to the disk. Sophisticated programs will stop data transmission output from the host computer with a "handshaking" signal, and then write the previously transmitted data to the disk. With handshaking, the buffer memory can be filled and emptied over and over, the only limitation being the space available on the disk. Since the 32,000 character memory size limit is only about 5 minutes of recording at 1200 baud, the ability to continuously save data on the disk is important. Different computers use different methods to stop and start data transmission. One method, Control-S/Control-Q handshaking, stops the host computer from sending data when a Control-S (ASCII code 19) is sent by the microcomputer and starts sending again after Control-Q (ASCII code 21) is received. When using handshaking, characters are sent to a buffer until it is filled. Once the buffer is full, the Control-S signal is sent to stop transmission. The text is then written to the disk. Then the Control-Q signal is sent to restart text transmission. Control-Q/Control-S handshaking is recognized by both of

CONNECTING HOME COMPUTER TO A MODEM

Figure 4 Schematic of cable for connecting home computer to a modem. Most of the common special control lines are connected.

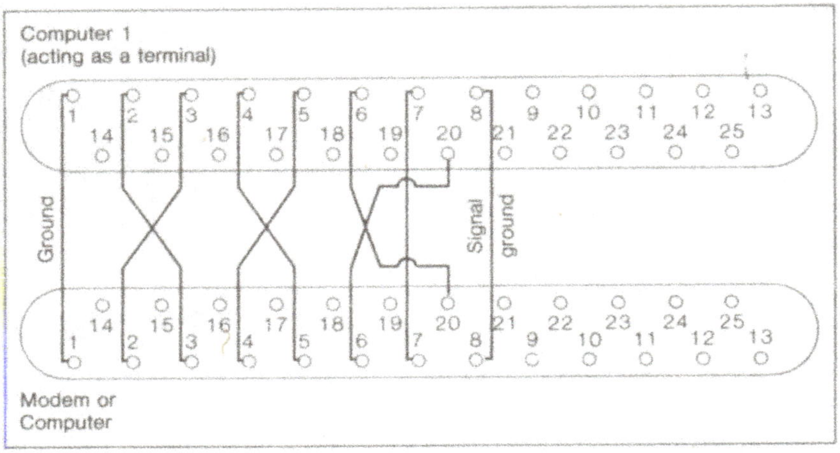

the major communications networks, Tymnet and Telenet,[6] and by the popular smaller networks, CompuServe and The Source.

A microcomputer program capable of sending data from the keyboard and displaying received data on the screen, and also of recording data on the disk using handshaking will satisfy 90% of your communications needs. Occasionally, however, you may want to send data to a host computer. For example, you might wish to send papers written with your word processor to a distant computer for printing or distribution. In the future you may be able to update patient records and send them to a hospital computer, or send billing information to an insurance company's computer.

Sending data from a microcomputer to another computer is nearly the inverse of receiving it. The data to be sent is read from the disk and stored in a memory buffer. Then it is sent to the host computer as if it had been typed at the keyboard.

[6] Control-Q/Control-S handshaking is also known as *flow control.* On Tymnet, special characters can be typed as you log in to enable flow control. On Telenet, the command FLOW ON is used.

However, sending data from memory buffer is different from sending keyboard characters to another terminal. Few people type faster than 100 words per minute (10 characters per second), and those who do can do it only in short bursts. Yet a computer with the slowest modem can transmit continuously at 300 words per minute without pausing for anything. Host computers not designed to receive text at such a rapid continuous rate will lose data, just as a microcomputer loses data without handshaking. Therefore, some host computers, including the Tymnet and Telenet mainframes, use Control-S/Control-Q handshaking (Telenet calls this handshaking T-Flow On) for input as well as output. Computers not using handshaking signals can manage to keep up if there are pauses at the end of each line. Some sophisticated communications programs are designed to actually slow down the normal communications speed. For example, such programs would send data at 30 char/sec (i.e., 0.033 sec/char) with a 0.067 second pause after each character, for an effective speed of 10 char/sec.

COMMUNICATION ERRORS

A communications program designed to make a microcomputer act like a simple terminal can be used with most computers. Using a microcomputer, however, is different from using a terminal. If you send or receive data on a terminal, you see exactly what was transmitted, and transmission errors ("noise" on the line) usually show up as unusual characters such as "PHY3ICIAN" or "198%." Thus, you have a chance to recognize the error at once and correct it. Programs that take data from another computer directly and put it on disk without review will record such errors along with the good data. These errors can be avoided entirely with proper error detecting/correcting protocols. Communications programs that use these protocols can detect transmission errors and ask the sending computer to retransmit the data.

For microcomputers, the most popular communication program with error corrections is MODEM-7. Developed by Ward Christensen for 8-bit microcomputers and recently extended to the 16-bit IBM-PC-like computers, MODEM-7 transmits data in "records" of 128 characters (bytes). Along with the data, it also sends an error check character called a "check sum." The receiving computer calculates the same check-sum from the 128 characters it receives. If the computed sum does not agree with the one transmitted, there was an error in transmission. A more sophisticated technique, the cyclic redundancy check (CRC), is based on the product of the ASCII codes of the text transmitted. In either case, when the receiving computer realizes there has been an error, it can ask for a retransmission of the record.

Error checking/detecting methods require that the communications running on both the sending and receiving computers use the same protocol (for practical purposes this means using compatible communication programs). Hobbyists have used the MODEM-7 protocol for several years because it is available for most microcomputers, often free or for only a small copying fee. The MODEM-7 protocol is also available in many commercial programs. CompuServe, a large time-sharing network, provides its own error-correcting protocol to users of the system.

Error detection/correction will become even more important in the future. If you plan to use your microcomputer for sending patient-related data to other computers, error-free transmission is especially important.

USING A COMMUNICATIONS PROGRAM

The fastest way to learn about computer-to-computer communications is to try it with one of the national information services. Radio Shack, for example, sells a package for $20 that enables you to call up CompuServe (5000 Arlington Centre Blvd., Columbus, OH 43220, (800) 848-8990) or Dow Jones Information Service for 1 hour free; additional time on CompuServe costs $5 per hour in the evenings (6:00 P.M.–5:00 A.M., local time). CompuServe has special interest sections so that people with similar computers or interests can exchange information and programs. One of these, sponsored by AAMSI (American Association of Medical Systems and Informatics), enables physicians to discuss computers and exchange solutions to medical computing problems.

Another way to start is to dial up a local Remote Bulletin Board System (RBBS) consisting of dial-up access microcomputers that hobbyists or computer stores have set up for exchanging messages and programs. Ask your local computer store to give you the telephone number of one of these systems. Once you gain access to a local system, you will find lists of other RBBS systems, and you can leave a message asking for further help. CompuServe or one of these local networks will put you in contact with technically sophisticated hobbyists who will readily share programs and information with you, and can give you expert advice on specific topics.

To do this, you need a communications program such as is described above. Many manufacturers now supply these programs with their units. For example, the IBM-PC comes with a simple communications program written in BASIC. Another program for the IBM-PC, PC-TALK[7], is available as part of the "Free-ware" program. You can copy PC-TALK from a friend (or from an IBM-RBBS system) and if you like it, send the author $35. Communications programs for the APPLE computer are available from Apple, and from D. C. Hayes, a company that sells a low speed modem that fits inside the Apple computer. Your Apple dealer can tell you about a nationwide network of Apple bulletin board systems. If you have a Radio Shack computer, you can get a communications program as part of the CompuServe package.

Computers with the CP/M operating system can use a descendent of the MODEM-7 program called MDM710. Versions of this program are available for most popular 8080 and Z80 computers, including the Heath-H89, Osborne-1, Kaypro, Northstar, Apple with Z80 Softcard, Televideo, Zenith-Z100, Xerox-820, and others. Different versions have been modified to work with a computer's specific communications chip. MDM710 is one of the most versatile microcomputer communications programs, and since it is in the public domain, it can be copied freely. It is available from the SIG/M national users group on a variety of different disk formats[8].

Commercial programs cost from $25 to $250. However, more expensive often does not imply better. Several expensive programs use proprietary communications protocols that require you to purchase two copies of the program (one for each computer), but do not support the more popular error-free MODEM-7 protocol. You should look at communications programs that:

1. Allow your computer to

MOST IMPORTANT RS232 SIGNALS

Table 1

	DB25P PLUG		DB25S SOCKET
	DATA TERMINAL EQUIPMENT		DATA COMMUNICATION EQUIPMENT
PIN#	FUNCTION	DIRECTION OF SIGNAL	FUNCTION
1	Protective ground	N/A	Protective ground
2	Transmit data	→	Receive data
3	Receive data	←	Transmit data
4	Request to send	→	
5		←	Clear to send
6		←	Data set ready
7	Signal ground	N/A	Signal ground
8		←	Carrier detect (modem has tone)
20	Data terminal ready	→	

[7]This program is described in *PC Magazine* (1982) 2(2): 413. In addition, *PC World* (1983) 1(5) is devoted to communications programs for the IBM-PC. PC-Talk III is available from Headlands Press, Inc., P.O. Box 862, Tiburon, CA 94920 for $35. If you send them two formatted disks and a self-addressed stamped envelope, they will send the program free.

send and receive all 127 ASCII characters (some preempt certain characters for control functions);

2. Communicate reliably at a speed of at least 1200 baud;

3. Allow recording of files larger than memory buffer by using handshaking;

4. Are capable of sending data from a file as if the data had been typed on the keyboard (usually line feed characters must be stripped from files, and handshaking or pauses may be necessary);

5. Support the MODEM-7 protocol for file transfer from bulletin board systems.

MAKING THE CONNECTION

Once you have a computer, an RS232 serial port, a modem and a communications program, you are ready to call up another computer. If you are using a program written for your computer, you will likely have no problems. Simply start up the program, set the communications speed (if necessary), and go into terminal mode. Then dial the phone number of the remote computer and wait for it to answer with a tone. If you are using a low speed modem, you will hear a high-pitched tone and your modem will respond with a lower-pitched tone. With a high speed modem, you will hear a mixture of tones. If you press keys before you make a telephone connection, you may not see anything on the screen because the characters are not echoed by the distant computer. After the computers are connected, however, the host computer will echo characters. Many host computers, including those of the network TYMNET and most microcomputer bulletin board systems, expect you to type a carriage return several times to determine the communications speed. Modems like

(Continued on page 86)

*SIG/M, Box 97, Iselin, NJ 08830. SIG/M distributes disks of public domain software for a small handling fee, usually $4 per disk. In addition, many local computer clubs also purchase the disks and make copies at meetings. You can write to SIG/M and find the address of the nearest local distribution point. Currently, they are distributing about 110 software disks for most popular computers.

AMERICAN STANDARD CODE FOR INFORMATION INTERCHANGE

Table 2 The ASCII code assigns numbers to 128 numbers, letters, punctuation and non-printing characters. The first 32 numbers are called "control characters." These characters do not print, but may have other special functions, such as carriage return, linefeed, or backspace.

Note that the numbers of the ASCII code naturally group in columns of 32. Control-M, or RETURN, is number 13, the letter "M" is 13 + 64 or 77, and lower case "m" is 77 + 32 or 109.

CONTROL CHARACTERS		NUMBERS AND PUNCTUATION		UPPER CASE LETTERS		LOWER CASE LETTERS	
CHAR	ASCII CODE	CHAR	ASCII CODE	CHAR	ASCII CODE	CHAR	ASCII CODE
NUL	0	SP	32	@	64	'	96
CTRL A	1	!	33	A	65	a	97
CTRL B	2	"	34	B	66	b	98
CTRL C	3	#	35	C	67	c	99
CTRL D	4	$	36	D	68	d	100
CTRL E	5	%	37	E	69	e	101
CTRL F	6	&	38	F	70	f	102
BELL	7	'	39	G	71	g	103
BKSP (backspace)	8	(	40	H	72	h	104
TAB	9	)	41	I	73	i	105
LNFEED (linefeed)	10	*	42	J	74	j	106
CTRL K	11	+	43	K	75	k	107
CTRL L (formfeed)	12	,	44	L	76	l	108
RETURN	13	–	45	M	77	m	109
CTRL N	14	.	46	N	78	n	110
CTRL O	15	/	47	O	79	o	111
CTRL P	16	0	48	P	80	p	112
CTRL Q	17	1	49	Q	81	q	113
CTRL R	18	2	50	R	82	r	114
CTRL S	19	3	51	S	83	s	115
CTRL T	20	4	52	T	84	t	116
CTRL U	21	5	53	U	85	u	117
CTRL V	22	6	54	V	86	v	118
CTRL W	23	7	55	W	87	w	119
CTRL X	24	8	56	X	88	x	120
CTRL Y	25	9	57	Y	89	y	121
CTRL Z (end of file)	26	:	58	Z	90	z	122
ESC (escape)	27	;	59	[	91	{	123
FS	28	<	60	\	92	¦	124
GS	29	=	61	]	93	}	125
RS	30	>	62	^	94	~	126
US	31	?	63	—	95	DEL (delete)	127

TROUBLESHOOTING

If your attempt to connect to a distant computer fails, it's time for detective work. Make sure everything is plugged in—power cords, telephone, cables. If you are dialing up a computer, you should hear a distinct tone and your modem should cause that tone to change when it connects. If you do not hear the tone, check the phone number. If the tone does not change, then check your modem. If you are using a high-speed modem to call a low-speed connection, the two modems may not connect. Change to a low-speed modem or try a high-speed connection.

Next, make sure you are using your modem program correctly. Most communications programs have two modes—terminal and command. In terminal mode, everything you type is sent to the modem. In command mode, typing goes to your microcomputer. Command mode sets the communications speed, upload or download files, and exit back to the operating system. To be sure you are using your modem program correctly, start it up, set the communications speed to 300 (low-speed modem) or 1200 baud, go into terminal mode, and press some keys. (These keys will probably not be echoed to the screen unless you are using an intelligent modem like the Hayes Smartmodem™.) Then type the character that allows you to return to command mode (Control-E for MDM710, ESCape with many other programs.) You should then be able to return to the operating system. If you have an intelligent modem and your typing is echoed, then everything is working properly and you can type the commands to dial the phone. You should then hear a dial tone; if you don't, the phone is probably not connected properly.

If you still have problems after going through the modem program, then your computer and modem are not properly connected, either because of a bad cable, bad interface, or faulty communications program. Most modems have a self-test, or half-duplex mode, sometimes called loop-back, that sends characters directly back to the computer when they are typed. To test your computer-modem connection, put the modem in half-duplex or echo mode and type some characters. If the characters appear on the screen, your connection is working and the trouble is probably in the modem-distant computer connection. If garbled characters appear, check the communications speed (baud rate) and the parity and word length settings on the RS232 interface port. Many modems also have a light that blinks when a character is received. If this light blinks, but characters are not displayed, you may have a problem with communications speed. Make sure your computer and communications program are set to communicate at the right speed (usually 300 or 1200 baud). If the characters are not echoed, check the interface, program, and cable by unplugging the cable from the modem. Using the null modem, plug it into something else (for example, a printer).

If you can send characters to the printer, but it prints other characters, the communications speed is probably wrong. If you can send characters to the printer without the null modem, then your cable wires may be switched.

If the above tactics have not solved your problem it is time to call for help. The remaining suggestions are only for true computer hobbyists. Try a male/female connector that reverses pins 2/3, 4/5, 6/20. On the other hand, the modem may require status signals, either Request To Send (pin 4) or Data Terminal Ready (pin 20). Check these signals with a voltmeter and compare your readings to the requirements listed in the modem specifications. If a status signal is required, make sure that the cable links the correct pins. If the cable is properly wired but the voltage reading is zero, then your computer may be unable to generate the necessary signal. Some modems require a voltage on pin 20 that can be found on another connector pin, often pin 6. If the modem seems to be receiving characters (because the light blinks), but characters do not appear on your screen, then your computer may require status signals such as Data Set Ready (pin 6).

By isolating the different parts of your computer-modem connection you should be able to locate the problem and substitute a different cable or modem. If all else fails, get your computer dealer to fix your computer's serial interface[9].

My descriptions of equipment and programs deal with the standard asynchronous communications used by most microcomputers and dial-up mainframe computers. Direct (nontelephone) linkages to many large computers (for example, IBM mainframes) require more expensive communication chips, modems, and software[10].

[9] For a more complete discussion of these problems, see *The Complete Handbook of Personal Computer Communications* by Alfred Glossbrenner, 1983, New York, St. Martin's Press.

[10] Two popular IBM communication protocols are BISYNC and SDLC. These methods require synchronization between the terminal and the computer. A group of data (often a line of text) is collected and sent as a block. The standard IBM-PC communications chips and most popular modems cannot process synchronous communications.

the Hayes Smartmodem™ will interpret commands, dial the telephone, and let you see characters on the screen as you press the keys. These characters are being echoed by the modem itself. When you dial the phone (using commands to the Smartmodem™) you will hear the host computer connect to the modem.

When everything is working, you will see a message after typing some characters and you are ready to explore the world of computer-to-computer communications.

TERMINAL EMULATION

Some computer communications programs offer a sophisticated feature called *terminal emulation.* This allows your microcomputer and terminal to act like another brand of terminal, for example, the Digital Equipment Corporation VT-100 terminal. Terminal emulation is used with computers like the IBM-PC and Apple, which have built-in memory-mapped video displays. If you only use your computer to download information from a larger computer, you do not need terminal emulation. It is frequently needed if you use your computer as a terminal for full screen editing programs running on the remote computer. It may also be needed to enter or display patient data, particularly if the host computer sends control characters for moving the cursor and erasing the screen. Most microcomputer bulletin boards, such as CompuServe and The Source, work without terminal emulation.

With everything working properly, you are ready to dial up one of the commercial networks like CompuServe or The Source, or your local RBBS network (do not be surprised if the line is frequently busy). Once you access your local RBBS you can get plenty of free software, including programs for cataloging disks, for modifying text editing systems, even some of the newer communications programs, not to mention computer games. If you dial up CompuServe, enter GO SFP-5 to access the Medical Computing SIG, and for a modest surcharge, you can get financial information by entering GO FIN-1. To access the special interest groups for any brand of computers, enter GO PCS-50. ("The Exchange" M.D. Computing, Vol. 1, No. 1.)

In this issue I have described how to connect your home computer to other computers over the telephone. In future issues, we will discuss how to connect computers within the office and how to set up computers so you can use them via telephone from outside.

SECURITY

Physicians considering converting their office computer to dial up access should be aware of the security problems involved. Once your computer is accessible over telephone lines, it is difficult to insure that you are the only one using it. Recently, for example, 10 chipheads (hackers, whiz-kids) inspired by the film *War Games* (in which a teenage computer whiz gains access to a Defense Department computer and almost triggers a nuclear war) gained access to a computer at our top secret nuclear weapons research laboratory, Los Alamos. These chipheads—ranging in age from 15 to 22—reached the lab's computer via a dial-up access from Minnesota. They were able to do this because Los Alamos has a computer connected to Telenet, a computer network available to the general public. (At Los Alamos, computers with sensitive information are not connected to the telephone network.) For now, the only way to ensure the security of your office computer is to keep it off the telephone network.

CONCLUSION

Enough talk. The time has come to call up a local computer and start typing. One of the bulletin boards, such as CompuServe, would be a good start. People ask for help on these boards. One of the most commonly asked questions is what kind of a computer or printer to buy. Reading responses to this question from other bulletin board users can be more more informative than a salesman's pitch.

PROGRAMMING LANGUAGES II

WILLIAM R. PEARSON, Ph.D.

Our first tutorial on programming languages [Bruce Blum's article in *M.D. COMPUTING*, Vol. 1, No. 5] discussed how the evolution of computer languages has made it easier to write programs. The earliest computers did not have programming languages per se. Instead, instructions were entered by toggling them in through control panels or by punching them onto paper tape. By the mid-1950s, the work of programmers had lightened a bit. Assembly language, a symbolic way of writing machine instructions, was in common use, and FORTRAN, the first high-level language, had been introduced. COBOL and ALGOL soon followed.

To review the features of these three early programming languages: FORTRAN made it easy to write scientific programs by providing a simple algebraic language for manipulating whole numbers (integers), real numbers (floating point), and arrays or matrices of numbers. COBOL was written for business data processing. COBOL statements resemble English, not algebra, and COBOL made it easy to manipulate "records" (variables that could hold several different kinds of information like an employee's name, social security number, and earnings). ALGOL, a scientific language, first introduced the block-structured control statements that are now available in most modern programming languages.

FORTRAN, COBOL, and ALGOL are just three examples of the programming languages available on many large mainframes and minicomputers. By the time microcomputers were introduced in the mid-'70s, dozens of computer languages had been introduced. You may recognize some of the names:

WILLIAM R. PEARSON, Ph.D.
William R. Pearson is an Assistant Professor of Biochemistry at the University of Virginia School of Medicine, Charlottesville. His research interests are in molecular biology and the control of gene expression in mammalian cells. He uses micro- and mainframe computers to study DNA and protein sequences, using programs written in FORTRAN, BASIC, PASCAL, and C.

ANY HIGH-LEVEL LANGUAGE REQUIRES A PROGRAM TO TRANSLATE IT INTO A FORM THE COMPUTER UNDERSTANDS.

APL, BASIC, BLISS, C, FORTH, LISP, LOGO, MUMPS, PL/I, RPG, SAIL, Smalltalk, SNOBOL. There was even a "happy" programming language called JOVIAL. It was one of the first, and is still used by the Defense Department. Each of these languages was developed for a specific reason: APL for concise descriptions of mathematical problems, FORTH for the interactive control of telescopes, MUMPS for medical record processing, SNOBOL for processing strings of text. In the last few years many applications packages, such as database systems, have developed their own "built-in" languages. For example, you can write programs in dBASE II, the popular database package for microcomputers.

Part 2 of this tutorial (in this issue) and Part 3 (in the next issue) describe many of the more popular programming languages for microcomputers. In addition to discussing the obvious differences among languages, we will try to give you their flavor and indicate their strengths and weaknesses.

With minicomputers and mainframes you usually have the choice of one version of FORTRAN, COBOL, or one of the other popular languages—the one offered by the machine's manufacturer. For microcomputers, the choices are much richer. Not only can you obtain almost any language, but you can choose from many versions of the same language. You have a choice of a dozen PASCALS, a half dozen C's, and at least three FORTRANS. You can use the BASIC interpreter that comes with the machine, buy another vendor's BASIC interpreter, or choose one of many BASIC compilers. Deciding to use a certain version of a computer language is not like choosing brands of rock salt. There are important differences in the compilation speed (the time it takes to translate language statements into machine-usable form), the execution speed (the time it takes to run the programs), the size of the compiled programs (the amount of memory required to run the programs), and the degree to which the languages adhere to the language standards (in case you want to run your program on different machines). Most microcomputer languages have limitations regarding the amount of data that can be stored or the size of the program that can be written. Finally, how the language is molded to the microcomputer can be as important as all of the other properties of the language itself.

BASIC, PASCAL, and C are the most popular microcomputer languages—with BASIC on the top because it usually comes with the computer and it is easy to use. When we talk about a computer language, we must distinguish the language (that is, its syntax and semantics) from its implementation (whether it is compiled or interpreted). A language can be implemented as a compiler (in a batch effort the entire program you've written is translated into instructions that can be executed by the computer) or as an interpreter (the computer retranslates the statements each time it encounters them). Whether a language is implemented as an interpreter or a compiler affects the speed of the computer's response and the ease or difficulty of editing a program.

BASIC is usually thought of as an interpreted language, but there are also compiled versions. PASCAL and C are traditionally compiled languages (though some versions now have interpreters). They are also the most popular languages for developing large programs on micros. A current controversy in language design, discussed later in this article, pits PASCAL, which has very strong typing, against C, which does not.

Before we discuss these languages, bear in mind: my advice is that most medical practitioners should not use any high-level language. Generally, your time would be better spent if you purchased a prewritten program. Most special tasks can be accommodated either by spreadsheet programs or database management programs. These may require some programming talent to use fully, but do not require the same expertise or effort as a standard programming language.

BASIC

BASIC, or Beginner's All-purpose Symbolic Instruction Code, was revolutionary in 1960, when it was written by John Kemeny and Thomas Kurtz for Dartmouth undergraduates. BASIC programs are similar to FORTRAN programs in many ways, but BASIC is much easier to learn and use. The language syntax is more uniform and simpler than FORTRAN, and it was implemented as an interpreter, which makes it easier to correct errors or change a line of the program. (This is one of the most striking differences between a compiler and an interpreter when you are writing a program.) At the time when BASIC was first being introduced, these differences were enormous.

When I learned FORTRAN in 1968 at the University of Illinois, writing a program required keypunching the program statements, then submitting the stack of cards to an operator and waiting two to six hours for a printout. Since I was learning keypunching, FORTRAN, and programming simultaneously, the only progress I made during the first four or five submissions was learning I had misspelled a word like SUBROUTINE or omitted a required comma. Had I been at Dartmouth using BASIC, I would have found these simple errors in seconds (because BASIC points out your errors as you type them in), and would have finished my computer work in hours instead of days. Thus, the biggest advantage of BASIC over FORTRAN has to do with its usual implementation as an interpreter, not the differences in the program statements. However, standard BASIC does provide a number of powerful and easy-to-use statements, such as text string manipulation, that are not available in standard FORTRAN.

Any high-level language requires a program (the compiler or interpreter program) that translates the language into something else the computer can understand. The archetypical compiler processes a complete program or subroutine after it has been created with a text processor or keypunch machine. Because it "sees" the whole program (or subroutine) at once, it can translate all the variable names into internal references which optimize the program flow. And, of course, the translation step is only done once. Consequently, programs created by compilers tend to run much faster than those created by interpreters. But the price you pay for this efficiency is that it takes longer to write the program. Every change in the program requires you to recompile the entire program (not just the changes). Thus the debugging cycle—find an error, correct it, test it—is lengthy.

The typical interpreter processes each program statement (usually a single line) as it is encountered. Most interpreters include an editor. As you type each program statement, the editor checks for typographical and syntax errors and reports them to you immediately. The statements you've typed can be run right away even when the program is not complete. Thus, you can change a statement and immediately test the program by running it. In addition, the interpreter can break into the execution of your program and examine the state of any of the program variables by name. This makes it much easier to find and correct program errors. The price you pay for this speed and flexibility in program development is that the finished program runs less efficiently than a compiled program—sometimes by a factor of ten.

INTERPRETER VERSUS COMPILER PROCEDURE

Figure 1. The example below contrasts interpreters and compilers in the classic case, looking at a FORTRAN compiler and a BASIC interpreter. The steps are as follows:

	FORTRAN	BASIC
Step 1	Type in the program using a text editor or word processor.	Start the BASIC interpreter, type in the program, and correct the errors as they return to you.
Step 2	Exit the text editor and run the compiler. If any mistakes are found, such as spelling errors, go back to step 1, correct them, and repeat step 2.	Not needed.
Step 3	Combine the output of the compiler with the FORTRAN library, which contains special subroutines needed to run a FORTRAN program by running a linker.	Not needed.
Step 4	Run the program. Subtle mistakes, such as writing **sum = x(i)** when you intended **sum + x(i)**, will show up at run time. Then go back to step 1 and repeat all four preceding steps to correct them.	Run the program. At this point, if you detect other errors, you only need to interrupt the program, check the variable contents to be sure you understand the problem, correct the lines, and say "run again."

In the past, languages were *either* interpreted (e.g., BASIC, APL, and LISP) or compiled (FORTRAN, PASCAL, C). Today the boundary is less clear because some languages, such as BASIC and PASCAL, have *both* interpreters and compilers. Morever, some new compilers (called incremental compilers) report your syntax errors as you type in the statements. Others have symbolic debuggers which let you interrupt program execution and look at the contents of variables by name—just like an interpreter. From the other direction, some interpreters employ precompilers which translate the source statements into a more efficient internal form as you type them in. (See Figure 1.)

Not only does the compiler take more steps, but each of these steps takes more time. The edit/compile/link/run process takes 2–10 minutes on a micro, depending upon the compiler and the length of the program. Each time a single line is changed, the entire process must be repeated. In an interpreter, a single line can be changed in a few seconds and the program is immediately ready to run. Since it might take five or ten repetitions of "modify, compile, link, and run" to get a 30–40 line program working, a program that could take an hour to write with a compiler would take minutes with an interpreter.

The disadvantage of interpreters is that programs written in interpreted languages usually run more slowly than compiled programs, because the process of immediate interpretation (or translation) also means that the interpreter sees only the statement it is currently working on. In our statistics program example presented below, a compiled version would run very fast because the additions in the FOR loop can be translated to just a few machine instructions. But a BASIC interpreter would have to retranslate each statement in the loop each time the loop was executed. Thus if N were 20 in the example, the compiled program would be translated once and executed 20 times, while the interpreted program would be translated 20 times and executed 20 times.

In theory, it is possible to obtain the best of both worlds. Develop your programs in the BASIC interpreter, and when they are running perfectly, use the compiler. MicroSoft makes both a BASIC interpreter and a compiler for CP/M and MS-DOS computers. The compiled programs usually run about ten times faster. However, there are practical barriers to this approach, because the syntax and features of the two versions differ in important ways.

How is BASIC different from FORTRAN? Let's again use an example which calculates the mean and standard deviation of a list of numbers. To save time, we can calculate the standard deviation of a list of numbers using the formula:

$$\text{S.D.} = \sqrt{\frac{\text{N} \times \text{SUMSQ} - \text{SUM} \times \text{SUM}}{\text{N} \times (\text{N}-1)}}$$

Figure 2 shows a shorter version of the sample FORTRAN program presented in part 1 of the tutorial *[see page 32 of this volume]*. Since our new formula accumulates the squares of the data rather than the difference between the data and the mean, will will use two "double precision" variables to avoid round-off errors. Our new program would be written in FOR-

STANDARD DEVIATION IN *FORTRAN*

Figure 2A

```
C       Calculate standard deviation of a list of numbers
C       FUNCTION STDDEV(X,N)
        DIMENSION X(1)
        DOUBLE PRECISION SUM, SUMSQ
C
C          initialize sum and sumsq
        SUM = 0.0
        SUMSQ = 0.0
C
C          calculate the sums
C
        DO 10 I = 1,N
        SUM = SUM + X(I)
     10 SUMSQ = SUMSQ + X(I)*X(I)
C
C       check if N = 1, if so, stddev = 0.0
C
        STDDEV = 0.0
        IF (N.GT.1) STDDEV = SQRT((N*SUMSQ-SUM*SUM)/(N*(N-1)))
        RETURN
        END
```

STANDARD DEVIATION IN *BASIC*

Figure 2B

```
100  REM Program for calculating mean and std.dev.
110  DIM X(100)
120  INPUT "How many numbers would you like to average?",N
130  IF N<=0 GOTO 120
140  FOR I = 1 TO N
150     PRINT I,
160     INPUT X(I)
170  NEXT I
180  REM All the numbers are in X(I), now add them up
185  REM (# below denotes double precision in BASIC)
200  SUM# = 0#
205  SUMSQ# = 0#
210  FOR I = 1 TO N
220     SUM# = SUM# + X(I)
225     SUMSQ# = SUMSQ# + X(I)*X(I)
230  NEXT I
240  MEAN = SUM#/N
250  IF (N<=1) THEN STDDEV = 0! ELSE
              STDDEV = SQR((N*SUMSQ# -
              SUM#*SUM#)/(N*(N-1)))
270  PRINT "Mean: ",MEAN," Std dev: ",STDDEV
```

TRAN as shown in Figure 2A. Figure 2B shows the same program written in BASIC.

As you can see, BASIC is very similar to FORTRAN. Several of the statements are identical, such as SUM = SUM + X(I), while others are very similar: FOR I = 1 TO N is similar in form and function to DO 10 I = 1,N. But there are some important differences.

The first obvious difference as you look at the BASIC and FORTRAN program examples is that all BASIC statements begin with line numbers (100, 110, . . .). BASIC requires line numbers, which its internal editor uses to help you correct a BASIC program. To correct a line, you need only retype it using its line number reference; to insert a line between 100 and 110, just number it 105. Obviously, the first thing you learn in BASIC is to number your lines in multiples of 5 or 10 so you can make insertions.

The other main difference between the BASIC and FORTRAN examples is that the BASIC example is complete. You could type it into your computer and it would run. The FORTRAN example is a subroutine, and must be incorporated into a larger main program. We discuss subroutines below.

BASIC programs manipulate the same kinds of data as FORTRAN programs—integers and real numbers. But BASIC can also manipulate text strings, a feature that makes it popular with business programmers who have to manipulate names, addresses, and other such text. A BASIC program can concatenate (add) text strings to form new text. For example:

```
[095  REM program to show text string
      concatenation]
 100  FIRSTN$ = "M.D."
 110  LASTN$ = "Computing"
 120  LASTFIRST$ = LASTN$ + "," +
      FIRSTN$
 130  LASTLAST$ = FIRSTN$ + " " +
      LASTN$
 140  PRINT FIRSTLAST$, LASTLAST$

      Computing, M.D.       M.D. Computing
```

In addition to handling integers, reals, and text strings, some BASICs also have matrix instructions which make it easier to add and multiply matrices and (in some systems) compute the determinant of a matrix. But BASIC does not have the more complicated record or structure data types of COBOL, PASCAL, and C, so that it is not possible to store an employee's name, social security number, and hourly wage in one variable and then manipulate them as a single entity.

THE REPEATED USE OF BASIC'S MISCHIEVOUS *GO TO* STATEMENT CAN LEAD TO SOME VERY TANGLED AND DIFFICULT-TO-DEBUG LOGIC FLOWS—OFTEN CALLED SPAGHETTI CODE.

The two major criticisms of BASIC as a language are that it does not have true subroutines and that it is missing statements such as "DO UNTIL" and "CASE" that permit good structuring of a program. A subroutine is a small program complete in itself that can take data passed from a larger program, process the data, and pass something back to the calling program. Subroutines also permit you to employ the strategy of "divide and conquer." You divide a larger project into the development of many small subroutines. It is much easier to write and debug many small programs than one large one. BASIC's GOSUB is similar to subroutines, but because it is not independent, it may not run when added to another program because you may have accidentally used the same variable name in the two programs.

Statements like "DO WHILE" and "CASE" found in more modern languages like PASCAL and C are program functions to control looping based on actual testing of the process, as opposed to the loop controls used in FORTRAN and BASIC which give an absolute numeric count of how many loops to make. These statements make it easier to understand what the program code is supposed to accomplish, and therefore easier to debug the program.

The absence of structured control statements requires the BASIC programmer to use the mischievous GO TO statement. GO TO statements force the program to jump away from the present location several statements or several pages ahead. Sometimes the program code in the new location includes another GO TO statement sending the logic to another distant location. This can lead to some very tangled, difficult-to-debug logic flows—often called spaghetti code.

These criticisms certainly apply to the most ubiquitous BASIC in computerdom—Microsoft BASIC. But they do not apply to all BASICs. In fact, the American National Standards Institute (ANSI) is currently reviewing a proposed standard for BASIC that includes subroutines, statements for program structuring and file management, and other optional capabilities for graphics and real-time applications [1]. There are many examples of BASICs with structuring and true subroutines. The computer BASICs supplied by Digital Equipment Corp. and Hewlett-Packard have many extensions, including considerable structuring, true subroutines, and other nonstandard commands. Digital Research's compiled BASIC, called CB80 for 8-bit computers and CB86 for 16-bit computers, has callable functions with capabilities similar to subroutines and a degree of structuring. Microsoft has a version of compiled BASIC called Business BASIC that has most of the capabilities of CB80. True BASIC and COSMOS's Revelation BASIC have separately compliable, callable subroutines, full structuring, and other attractive features for application development.

PASCAL

While BASIC is the most popular language for microcomputers, many computer scientists do not recommend it, and today most large computer projects will use either PASCAL or C. Indeed, some computer scientists have written that a student exposed to BASIC may be hopelessly brainwashed. These writers may be given to hyperbole; but there is more to programming, especially professional programming, than standard BASIC would indicate.

PASCAL was designed as a language for teaching students good programming practices. The first working compiler was produced in 1970, and the standard reference for PASCAL programs was published in 1974. Since then, more and more introductory computer science courses stress PASCAL rather than FORTRAN or BASIC. PASCAL was also designed to make it easy to write programs that could be proven correct—an important issue. At the time PASCAL was developed, software products were getting larger and costing more, but were temperamental and failure-prone. In fact, in 1971 it was quite common for systems to "crash" once a day because of a serious software failure. The situation has improved greatly since then because of the emphasis on correct programming.

Earlier research discovered that proving a program correct required it to have well-structured control statements and data structures. Without fully discussing what structuring means to programs, in general, good structuring implies that the program has a linear flow from the first to the last line, and that logic and data structures are organized hierarchically. A corollary is that GO TO's should be used rarely, or not at all, because they create logical tangles in program flow.

Data is structured by defining classes or types of data. One of the most common programming errors is not distinguishing between classes of data—like trying to add apples and oranges. If apples are represented by an integer number, and oranges are also represented by an integer, the compiler cannot know that this statement doesn't make sense:

```
total apples = delicious + valencia
total oranges = navel + mcintosh
```

PASCAL AND RECORD VARIABLES

Figure 3

```
type employee_record = record
        name : string[80];
        ssn : string[11];
        salary : real;
        hours : real;
    end;
  var employee ARRAY [1..1000] of employee_record;
—and then refer to a name as:
  writeln(employee[i].name);
```

The solution provided by PASCAL—and other "strongly typed" languages—is to declare the type of a variable explicitly, as in:

```
type
    apples = integer;
    oranges = integer;
var
    valencia, navel, mandarin: oranges;
    delicious, pippin, mcintosh: apples;
```

Since the compiler knows the apples are different from oranges (even though they are both represented by integer numbers), it can detect and forbid errors which mix variables. Using a strongly typed language allows the compiler to catch many errors before the program is ever run. PASCAL requires explicit use of variables and can more easily identify nonsensical statements. FORTRAN and BASIC do not offer this protection because they lack strong typing.

In addition to strong typing and a complete set of well-structured control statements (IF THEN ELSE, WHILE DO, REPEAT UNTIL, FOR), PASCAL has RECORD variables, variables which can hold several different kinds of data. For example, you can declare an array of employee information with the form shown in Figure 3. Our statistics example, written in PASCAL, is shown in Figure 4.

As you can see, PASCAL is a block-structured language like ALGOL. In addition, like ALGOL, PASCAL uses ":=" instead of "=" for assignment. This notation is designed to distinguish between the action of assignment—the process of storing the contents of the variable on the right side of the ":=" into the variable recorded on the left side—from the logical test to see if two items are the same. Note also that in the FORTRAN and BASIC programs, we did not have to do anything special to multiply or divide the integer "N" and the real numbers "SUMSQ". Since PASCAL is designed to protect against using different types of variables in arithmetic expressions, the integer must be explicitly converted to a floating point number. BASIC and FORTRAN do this automatically. (Though standard PASCAL does not provide a double-precision TYPE REAL, several microcomputer implementations do, as an extension.)

Programming languages, like human languages, shape the way we think about things. A powerful language like PASCAL makes it much easier to employ sophisticated methods to solve problems. That is why some computer scientists decry teaching BASIC. A student who has learned only BASIC may have less chance to devise inventive solutions to programming problems.

The introduction of PASCAL shifted the focus of introductory computer science courses from simply making a program compile to really learning something about solving programming problems. Computer textbooks shifted from sets of rules—teaching, for instance, that statement numbers could only be typed in the first five columns (as required by FORTRAN)—to essays on how to write programs using the best algorithms available. In a sense, programming courses evolved from grammar to literature.

Unfortunately, PASCAL is not without its faults. Since it was designed as an introductory teaching language, several features needed by working programmers were left out. Like many languages, PASCAL has very few input/output statements. The standard describes how to read lines or write lines, but there is no explicit provision for many kinds of file manipulations, such as jumping into the middle of a file and pulling out information, as needed in business applications. While PASCAL encourages subroutines because they make it easier to write well-structured programs, the language makes it difficult to use subroutine libraries. In the example above, the size of the array "x" was declared to be 100 numbers. A subroutine for 10 numbers requires a different program, as does a subroutine for 1000. And a subroutine to calculate the cost of apples must be different from one for oranges. PASCAL can also be annoying. In addition to the confusion between "=" and ":=", PASCAL requires that all statements end with a ";". Since IF () THEN ELSE" is considered a single statement, a ";" after the expression "stddev := 0" in our PASCAL programming example (Figure 4) would be an error because it would incorrectly signal the end of a statement.

PASCAL users and manufacturers soon became aware of these limitations. Since the microcomputer industry needed powerful compilers to meet the demand for new applications programs, compilers were written with extensions to supply the functions left out of the initial PASCAL specification. Unfortunately, each compiler writer put in different extensions, in an effort to make his product more powerful and thus more successful commercially. So while there are PASCAL compilers available for micros, minis, and mainframe computers, a program written with one PASCAL compiler usually must be modified extensively to work with another PASCAL because they use different extensions. One solution to this problem is to write programs which only use "standard" PASCAL, but the features which the standard lacks are so important that PASCAL without extensions is not a very useful language.

STANDARD DEVIATION IN *PASCAL*

Figure 4

```
FUNCTION stddev( x: ARRAY [1..100] OF REAL, n: INTEGER): REAL;
VAR
   i : integer;
   sum, sumsq : real;
BEGIN
   sum := 0;
   sumsq := 0;
   FOR i := 1 TO n DO
      BEGIN
         sum := sum + x[i];
         sumsq := sumsq + x[i]*x[i];
      END;
   IF (n < 1) THEN stddev := 0
   ELSE
   stddev := sqrt((FLOAT(n)*sumsq - sum*sum)/FLOAT(n*(n - 1)));
END {stddev}
```

A Quick Survey of PASCAL Compilers

Despite the differences in PASCAL compilers, there are some de facto standards. In the late 1970s, the computer science department at the University of California, San Diego, decided that it was cheaper to teach students using individual microcomputers than have a large number of students on a mainframe. At that time, the microcomputer market was just developing (the TRS-80 was not yet available), and no one microprocessor chip dominated. They designed a portable system which could be moved easily from one computer type to another. This was done by developing the compiler, editor, and teaching tools for an imaginary computer, and then writing a small program for the real microcomputer to make it act like the imaginary one. The package became available as UCSD PASCAL, and is currently sold and supported by SofTech Microsystems. An early version of UCSD PASCAL is used for Apple PASCAL. The package is also available for a very large number of other machines, including the 8080/Z80 computers, the IBM-PC and look-alikes, and even the extinct TI 99/4A. Since UCSD PASCAL is one of the most popular PASCAL compilers, many other compiler writers have used the same extensions.

The UCSD P-system marketed by SofTech is expensive, $500 to $700, and I do not recommend it for most computers. However, on the Apple and TI 99/4A, UCSD PASCAL is the only PASCAL compiler available, and the manufacturer sells it at a more modest price.

On the plus side, UCSD PASCAL is a microcomputer standard, and compilers are available for many different computers. But the P-system PASCAL compiler requires its own operating system, which is not compatible with the more popular CP/M or PC-DOS. So the P-system does not let you use popular text editors (like WordStar), communications programs, or other programming languages (FORTRAN is available, but not C). In addition, because programs are compiled into a machine language for an imaginary computer, and then interpreted by the actual computer running the program, P-system programs are usually five to ten times slower than programs compiled for the "native" machine.

There are several excellent PASCAL compilers available for both CP/M and PC-DOS, however. An exceptional buy among the group is Turbo-Pascal, from Borland Systems, for $49.95; it is available for both CP/M and PC-DOS. This compiler also comes with a WordStar-like text editor so that when the compiler finds an error, it can start up the text editor and display the mistake on the screen for you to fix. Turbo-Pascal seems to be a combination interpreter/compiler, so compilation is very fast. If you just want to get a taste of PASCAL, you can't beat the price. I have not used Turbo-Pascal, but I have used two other compilers, Pascal MT+ from Digital Research (for CP/M on 8080/Z-80 computers) and Microsoft Pascal (version 3 for MS-DOS and IBM-PC-like computers). Both cost about $300. I have used these compilers for transferring PASCAL programs running on other computers, and they worked well. The Microsoft PASCAL compiler offers a large number of extensions for sophisticated systems programming, and it is also compatible with both the original PASCAL standard and UCSD PASCAL.

STANDARD DEVIATION IN C

Figure 5

```
double stddev(x,n)
      float x; int n;
{
      double sum, sumsq;
      double sd;
      int i;
      for (sum = 0.0, sumsq = 0.0, i = 0; i<n; i++) {
            sum += x[i];
            sumsq += x[i] * x[i];
            }
      if (n>1) sd = sqrt((n*sumsq - sum*sum)/(n*(n-1)));
      else sd = 0;
      return sd;
      }
```

SYSTEMS PROGRAMMING LANGUAGES

FORTRAN, COBOL, ALGOL, BASIC, and PASCAL are programming languages for applications such as reconstructing an X-ray image, writing paychecks, or describing algorithms. Systems programs are another class of programs—the ones that form an operating system. They are used to type the contents of a file, list the files on a disk, or delete a file. Compilers, such as a FORTRAN or PASCAL compiler, are also systems programs.

Until the late '60s, systems programs were usually written in assembly language. Although systems programs use the same machine instructions as FORTRAN or COBOL programs, it was believed that only assembly language could provide the efficiency required by systems programs. And the popular high-level languages, FORTRAN and COBOL, were designed for specific applications that did not include text editors and compilers. There were several notable exceptions. In 1964, Burroughs introduced the B5500, a computer whose machine language was an ALGOL variant. At about the same time, the MULTICS operating system was written at M.I.T. in PL/I (a high-level language combining features of both FORTRAN and COBOL) for General Electric and Honeywell. Neither one of these systems was commercially successful, and it was not until ten years later that the UNIX operating system, written in a language called "C," demonstrated that an operating system could be written in a high-level language and be successful. Since then, the complexity of modern operating systems and the demand for reliable software has forced programmers to use high-level languages more for systems programming.

Although UNIX was written originally for research laboratory program development and only recently has been supported by computer manufacturers, some say it is the de facto standard for the new generation of 16- and 32-bit multiuser computers. While its popularity is based on its clean design, another benefit is that it is easy to implement UNIX on different computers since the operating system itself is written in C. UNIX has been implemented on computers ranging from a $7,000 Radio Shack Model 16 microcomputer to multimillion-dollar IBM mainframes.

C

How is a systems programming language like C different from other computer languages? While FORTRAN makes it easy to manipulate arrays of floating-point numbers, C is designed to manipulate bytes and words, the simplest units of working storage in a computer. In addition to the standard integer and floating-point data types, C programmers can manipulate unsigned integers, character or byte variables, pointers to other variables or a specific computer's memory locations, and structures made up of combinations of all of these types of data. Systems programmers can design efficient programs using "bit-fiddling" instructions usually only available in assembly language. In addition, C uses a complete set of flow control statements and recursion, providing a block structure similar to ALGOL or PASCAL. The statistics example could be written in C as shown in Figure 5.

The *for* statement shown is similar to the FORTRAN "DO" statement with a few extras. In FORTRAN, one can only initialize one variable, the index (I) in a DO statement. In the *for* statement, we set three variables, *sum*, *sumsq*, and *i* equal to 0. This ability to combine several assignments in the *for* loop helps make it clear that *sum* and *sumsq* must be set to zero before the loop starts. The "++" notation means to increment the preceding variable by one ("i++" is equivalent to "i = i+1"), and is just one of the ways C lets you take advantage of the computer's machine instructions (most computers have a special machine instruction for incrementing a variable by one). "sum += x[i]" is another example of C shorthand, and means "sum = sum + x[i]". Since statements of this form ("x = x+10" or "y = 3 * y") are very common in computer programs, this operator makes it easier for the compiler to translate such statements into efficient machine code.

The example also shows one of C's quirks. In all the other examples, the DO loop or *for* statement indexed *i* from 1 to *n*. In C the convention is different; arrays are indexed from 0 to *n*−1, and the *for* statement reads "for (i=0; i<n, . . .)". That means that when you declare an array of 100 elements they are numbered from 0 to 99; there is no element number 100.

C was developed at about the same time as PASCAL, and shares many of its features: a complete set of well-structured control statements (*if - else, while, for, repeat*) and a variety of data types, including structures which are similar to PASCAL's RECORD variables. But C and PASCAL are very different languages. The differences are due to the divergent philosophies behind the languages, and the functions the languages have served. PASCAL was designed as a teaching language to demonstrate and enforce the principles of structured programming. C was designed as a production language. The first C compiler was written so that an early version of the UNIX operating system (which was first written in assembly language) could be converted into a high-level programming language. While PASCAL was widely used for teaching programming within a few years after its introduction, very few C compilers existed outside the UNIX operating system until recently. Because C had more than six years to mature in the UNIX environment, C compilers are not plagued with extensions, and they adhere very closely to the UNIX standard. In the past several months, several colleagues and I have been developing a C program for studying protein evolution. This program has been compiled on four different computers (including an IBM-PC) and under three operating systems with virtually no changes.

GENERAL-PURPOSE LANGUAGES CAN BE USED FOR ACCOUNTING, TEXT EDITING, DATA REDUCTION, AND MORE.

C also has critics. Although the language has PASCAL-like control statements and structured data types, C makes no effort to enforce good programming practices. It is easy to write programming statements in C that are almost unreadable. For example, the loop of the statistics program could have been written as:

```
for
    sum = sumsq = 0.0, i = 0; i<n;
    sum + = *x, sumsq + = *x * *x,
    x + + , i + + ;
```

This form is much more difficult to follow. As a result, C has been referred to as a low-level language or structured assembly language. In addition, while many C programs are used for text editing and formatting, C does not have a string variable type, as do BASIC and PASCAL. C also makes heavy use of "pointers," variables which contain references to locations where data is stored instead of actual data. With pointers it is very easy to make serious mistakes, in which incorrect programs destroy data in other programs or in parts of the operating system. A recent manual for a Lattice C compiler for the IBM-PC warns that one user managed to destroy a memory copy of the directory for his hard disk drive with an incorrect pointer reference, thus effectively erasing all of the files on the drive. PASCAL keeps pointers on a much tighter rein because they are so dangerous. C also has several other features which make it easy to write a program which looks correct but in fact is not. For that reason, some C programs can be very difficult to debug.

Because C is such a simple, powerful language, and because more and more computer science students are being exposed to UNIX, C has become very popular. C compilers are available for CP/M and MS-DOS computers with prices ranging from $40 to $800, and compilers are also available for the Apple, Atari, and Radio Shack Color computers. The most popular C compiler for CP/M-based microcomputers is BDS C, which costs about $150. Although BDS C does not strictly conform to the UNIX standard for some file input/output functions, it is popular because it compiles programs very quickly, and because there is a vast array of public-domain software available for it. The fast compilation speed of BDS C can easily save thirty minutes to an hour in debugging a modest-sized program; the large number of compatible programs makes it easy to learn C by reading other people's code.

The $40 C compiler from Software Toolworks is also very good; it conforms closely to the UNIX standard input/output functions, but it takes much longer (minutes instead of tens of seconds) to compile programs. Neither of these compilers provides for manipulation of floating-point or real numbers. A subroutine package is available for the BDS C compiler, and floating-point functions can be added to the Software Toolworks compiler for an additional $30. Many microcomputer C compilers lack floating-point variables; many C programs are used for text processing, which requires only integer and character variables. The most expensive CP/M C compiler, the Whitesmith's compiler at $600, does provide floating point, but the program is very large and extremely slow.

Several C compilers for the new 16-bit IBM-PC-like computers are excellent. I use the Lattice C compiler ($500), but the CI-86 and DeSmet compilers ($350, $150) are also very good. All three compilers support the full UNIX C language, including "floats" and "longs." These three compilers also provide excellent support for the 8087 floating-point chip available for

IBM-compatible computers. This chip can speed up floating-point multiplication and division twentyfold.

OBTAINING COMPILERS

I recommend buying compilers by mail order. Paying list price for a spreadsheet or word processing program at your local computer store may make sense if they can help you use the program. But most computer stores don't carry many PASCAL or C compilers, and they won't be able to help you with programming. One excellent source for programs and advice is:

The Programmer's Shop
908 Providence Highway
Dedham, MA 02026
617/461-0120

They sell the BDS, Lattice, CI-86, and DeSmet C compilers, the Microsoft BASIC, FORTRAN, and PASCAL compilers, and the Digital Research FORTRAN, PASCAL, C, and CBASIC compilers, as well as many others.

Another excellent source for compilers for the IBM-PC and other MS-DOS-compatible machines is:

MicroWay
P.O. Box 79
Kingston, MA 02364
617/746-7341

Lastly, you should be aware of

Lifeboat Associates
1651 Third Avenue
New York, NY 10128
800/847-7078
212/860-0300

—the one central source for all software. They sell any program for any computer; but they charge list prices.

CONCLUDING REMARKS

In this tutorial we covered the three most popular programming languages for microcomputers: BASIC, PASCAL, and C. All three are general-purpose programming languages; you can use them for writing programs ranging from accounting to data reduction to word processing.

In the final segment (in a forthcoming issue of *M.D. COMPUTING*) we will discuss some more specialized languages (APL, FORTH, LISP, LOGO, Smalltalk, MUMPS) that have been developed to do one function—or just a few—very well. Often these languages provide built-in features that can cut programming time by a factor of ten. In addition, we will discuss some things to consider when choosing a programming language or compiler. □

REFERENCE

1. Anderson R. The proposed ANSI BASIC Standard. Byte 1983 (Feb):194–9.

BIBLIOGRAPHY

Books on computer programming have replaced car repair manuals and cookbooks in many bookstores, but quality has not always kept up with quantity. Two kinds of books are available for most languages. One is a textbook on programming that teaches more about programming than about the language. The second is a reference manual that describes exactly what language constructions are legal, but tells nothing about how to solve a particular problem. In the list below, ***Basic and the Personal Computer*** and ***Algorithms + Data Structures = Programs*** are examples of textbooks; ***The C Programming Language*** and ***Pascal: User Manual and Report*** are examples of reference manuals. Once you have learned one programming language, it is usually easy to move to other similar languages (BASIC, C, FORTRAN, PASCAL) with just a reference manual. Other languages, like APL, FORTH, and LISP (to be introduced in the next installment of this tutorial), may require more help.

BASIC

BASIC and the Personal Computer by Thomas Dwyer and Margot Critchfield, Addison-Wesley, 1978. This is a good general book on BASIC and includes an interesting variety of problems. The authors have written several other books for specific computers that I don't like as much.

C

The C Programming Language by Brian Kernighan and Dennis Ritchie, Prentice-Hall, 1978. This is THE standard book on C. Many manufacturers include it with their compilers. Kernighan has written several books on good programming practices, and Ritchie was one of the original authors of the UNIX timesharing system and the C language.

Several of the current CP/M C compilers are based on the Small C compiler written by Ron Cain and published in ***Dr. Dobbs' Journal*** several years ago. James E. Hendrix has made improvements in the compiler and published a detailed description in ***The Small C Handbook,*** Reston Publishing Co., Reston, VA (Prentice-Hall). The Small C compiler is written in C, so the book provides extensive examples of C programming as well as how a compiler actually works.

C Notes: A Guide to the C Programming Language by C. T. Zahn, Yourdon Press, New York, provides a good tutorial on how to use C's more powerful features.

PASCAL

An excellent advanced text on programming that uses PASCAL for its examples is ***Algorithms + Data Structures = Programs*** by Niklaus Wirth, Prentice-Hall, 1976. There are many more elementary PASCAL texts. If you are going to start learning programming with PASCAL use a text chosen for your particular computer and compiler. The Wirth book can be a second text on programming. The standard for the language is ***PASCAL: User Manual and Report*** by Kathleen Jensen and Niklaus Wirth, Springer-Verlag, 1978. This book tells you what you can do in PASCAL but not how to do it.

If you would like to take a quick look at a large number of languages running one program, look up "Eratosthenes Revisited: Once More Through the Sieve," by Jim and Gary Gilbreath, ***Byte,*** January, 1983, pp. 283–326. The authors compare BASICs, Cs, PASCALs, FORTHs, and many other languages running a simple program to calculate prime numbers. A sample program listing is presented for each programming language.

SOFTWARE SOURCES

B. D. Software
P.O. Box 2368
Cambridge, MA 02238
617/576-3828
BDS C compiler for CP/M, $150.

Borland International
4113 Scotts Valley Drive
Scotts Valley, CA 95066
800/227-2400 x953
408/438-8400
Turbo-Pascal for CP/M and MS-DOS, $49.95.

C-Ware Corp
P.O. Box 710097
San Jose, CA 95171
408/736-6905
DeSmet C and a debugging package, $150.

Computer Innovations
980 Shrewsbury Avenue
Suite J-507
Tinton Falls, NJ 07724
800/922-0169
201/542-5920
CI-86 C compiler for MS-DOS and CP/M-86, $395.

COSMOS Incorporated
19530 Pacific Highway South
Suite 102
Seattle, WA 98188
206/824-9942

Digital Research
160 Central Avenue
Pacific Grove, CA 93950
800/227-1617 x400
408/649-3896
FORTRAN 77, CBASIC, PASCAL MT+, COBOL, PL/I, C.

Lattice, Inc.
P.O. Box 3072
Glen Ellyn, IL 60138
312/858-7950
Lattice C compiler for MS-DOS and CP/M-86, $500.

Microsoft Corporation
10700 Northup Way
Bellevue, WA 98004
800/426-9400
PASCAL, FORTRAN, C, Business BASIC, BASIC for CP/M and MS-DOS (PC-DOS).

The Software Toolworks
15233 Ventura Boulevard
Suite 1118
Sherman Oaks, CA 91403
818/986-4885
C/80 compiler for CP/M, $49.95.

True BASIC, Inc.
39 South Main Street
Hanover, NH 03755
603/643-3882
Integrated package, $140.

PROGRAMMING LANGUAGES III

WILLIAM R. PEARSON, Ph.D.

In our last installment, we looked at three of the most popular languages used on microcomputers, BASIC, PASCAL, and C. BASIC, a direct descendant of FORTRAN, is easy to learn and quick to program in because it is implemented with an interpreter. PASCAL is a descendant of ALGOL, but it offers more powerful methods for specifying exactly how variables can be used, making it easier to write correct programs. Since BASIC was invented to teach introductory programming more easily (by providing a time-shared interpreter), it shares many of the shortcomings of the languages that preceded it (such as FORTRAN). PASCAL was introduced to correct problems with introductory languages; it is a powerful language, but it lacks features needed for real-world programming. "C" is a systems programming language that was used to develop UNIX; it has the structural features of PASCAL but few safeguards against mistakes.

In this final installment, we will look at some less well known languages available for microcomputers. Some, like PL/I, Modula II, and ADA, were developed to correct problems with earlier languages, such as FORTRAN and PASCAL. These languages look a lot like their parents: they have simple assignment statements (x = y * z), FOR loops, IF THEN ELSE, and so on. At the same time, other languages were developed for specific tasks. If you can read FORTRAN or PASCAL, it's easy to pick up C, ADA, PL/I, BASIC, or Modula II. But APL, FORTH, LISP, and MUMPS are so different that they are often unintelligible.

WILLIAM R. PEARSON, Ph.D.
William R. Pearson is an Assistant Professor of Biochemistry at the University of Virginia School of Medicine, Charlottesville. His research interests are in molecular biology and the control of gene expression in mammalian cells. He uses micro- and mainframe computers to study DNA and protein sequences, using programs written in FORTRAN, BASIC, PASCAL, and C.

PL/I

My first course in programming presented two languages, FORTRAN and PL/I. At that time (1968), PL/I was a newcomer compared to FORTRAN and COBOL, and it seemed to fill a niche halfway between them. Like FORTRAN, it had DO loops, subroutines, and floating-point arithmetic, but like COBOL, it had structured variables that could hold name, social security number, and pay records. In fact, PL/I seemed to have everything: you could play engineer and use scientific notation, or you could play accountant and use fixed-point arithmetic, or both. As a result, the PL/I compiler was very big, and it generated big, inefficient programs. PL/I was developed by IBM, and only IBM and a few other mainframe manufacturers offered it.

Although PL/I in its original form was unwieldy, it met the need for a powerful, structured programming language. In the mid-'70s, a subset of PL/I was developed that had most of the features and less of the frills. This language, PL/I subset G, is an ANSI (American National Standards Institute) standard language, and compilers are available for a wide range of minicomputers, including the DEC PDP-11 and VAX, Data General Eclipse, and Prime computers. In addition, Digital Research has developed PL/I compilers for both 8-bit and 16-bit microcomputers running CP/M, CP/M-86, and MS-DOS. PL/I is a powerful and versatile language. It is an excellent choice for software developers writing accounting programs for a large number of different mini- and microcomputers. But if you want to get something done in your home or office, PL/I is still probably too big. PASCAL and C are easier to learn, and because they are so popular, there are better compilers and textbooks available.

LOGO AND SMALLTALK ARE POWERFUL LANGUAGES BECAUSE THEY PROVIDE FUNCTIONS FOR MANIPULATING GENERAL LISTS OF SYMBOLS, AND NOT JUST TRADITIONAL NUMBERS AND TEXT.

MODULA II AND ADA

The creator of PASCAL, Niklaus Wirth, has developed a new language, Modula II, which eliminates most of PASCAL's shortcomings. Modula II has a number of features for developing systems software. Like C, it lets you manipulate system registers and implement instructions in a way similar to assembly language, as well as develop subroutine libraries and flexible subroutines. Modula II is just becoming available; unfortunately, it seems to share the PASCAL philosophy that the compiler knows more about your program than you do. This may be the case in the early stages of learning to program, but more advanced programmers may find Modula II getting in the way, rather than helping. Nonetheless, it is quite possible that Modula II will replace PASCAL for both teaching and practicing programming in the years ahead.

ADA is a language designed for most of the future programming by the Department of Defense. The language evolved through a series of competitions. At first glance, it appears very similar to PASCAL, with a large number of extensions for dealing with real-time programming, blips on a radar screen, targeting rockets, etc. But it is a much larger and more complicated language, and one researcher has warned that its complexity makes it dangerous for controlling refineries or nuclear weapons. It is so complicated that ADA compilers are just becoming available, running on very large machines. Since COBOL was also designed for the military and has become the most important language commercially, many have argued that ADA is the language of the future. But COBOL was designed at a time when there were very few high-level languages. ADA will be up against a lot more competition.

OTHER LANGUAGES

There are more than a dozen languages available for microcomputers, each with its own disciples. Here is a quick list, with comments.

APL

APL, A Programming Language, was developed in the mid-1960s by Kenneth Iverson at IBM. Dr. Iverson, a mathematician, wanted to write computer programs with the same concise notation and ease that he could describe mathematical problems. APL is a very powerful interpreted language, with many built-in functions. It is also very terse, and requires an unusual character set to denote these many functions. A statistics program could be written with just a few special characters in APL. Unfortunately, the language is so terse and powerful that sometimes it is almost impossible to read other people's programs, and difficult to read your own after a few weeks. APL proponents point out that the language is so powerful that it's easier to rewrite a program than to decipher one.

FORTH

FORTH was designed in 1969 to program the minicomputers controlling radio telescopes. Since these computers had limited memory and storage capability, FORTH was designed to be very compact, but also very efficient. FORTH is a kind of interpreter that includes its own compiler. FORTH programs are based on reverse polish notation (RPN), a way of representing mathematical equations popularized by the Hewlett-Packard calculator. Rather than typing A = B + C, one writes B C + A =. This is an especially efficient notation for the computer. With practice you can learn to read equations written in RPN almost as easily as in the conventional format. But arrays, IF statements, and DO loops written in RPN can be very obscure. Moreover, most FORTH implementations provide neither floating-point numbers nor structured or record data types. FORTH was designed to be simple and fast. FORTH programming can be very productive, but, as with APL, programs can be very difficult to understand. Many FORTH languages come with their own operating systems, like the UCSD P-system, and are not compatible with other programs for the computer. Inexpensive versions of FORTH are available for most small computers. Several are available from the FORTH Interest Group (FIG). FORTH was one of the first programming languages available for the Macintosh computer.

LISP, LOGO, and Smalltalk

All the programming languages we have discussed so far are designed to manipulate numbers and text. LISP, the most popular language for artificial intelligence programming, is used to manipulate ideas and solve problems. [See

"An Introduction to Lisp," by Walker and Blum, *[Chapter 16 of this volume]*. Several programs for medical diagnosis, including MYCIN for diagnosis of bacterial infection, are written in LISP. Programmers accustomed to the algebra-like statements of FORTRAN and BASIC find LISP expressions, which are based on a formalism from mathematical logic, very confusing. LISP, for LISt Processing, can manipulate lists of anything: numbers, words, diseases, symptoms, nouns, verbs, symbols, properties, deductions, and LISP statements. LISP provides an exceptionally good example of how a language can shape the way we think about problems. Many arithmetic expressions and traditional program control statements look strange written in LISP, but the movement and manipulation of complex data structures are natural. For example, note that the statement

```
(SETQ 'X (PLUS 'A 10))
```

is equivalent to X = A + 10, but the statement

```
(CAR (CDR (
   (DELICIOUS (WASHINGTON OREGON
   CALIFORNIA))
   (PIPPIN (NEWYORK MICHIGAN)) )))
```

—which extracts (PIPPIN)—does not have a simple equivalent.

I have several textbooks on LISP that describe it as a simple language. My experience has been limited, but I have always found it difficult to read or write LISP programs. If you want to learn LISP, there are LISP interpreters available for computers such as Apple, IBM-PC, and CP/M-based systems. The Software Toolworks sells a LISP interpreter, with several sample programs (including Eliza, the famous program that mimics psychotherapy), for $40.

While LISP is not the language for everyone, a "derivative" language, LOGO, may be. LOGO was developed at M.I.T. by Seymour Papert as a language for children—not so much to teach them programming or "computer literacy," but to help them learn how to solve problems. Papert studied with the developmental psychologist Jean Piaget, and designed LOGO to make it easier for children to develop mental models, and thus to learn. LOGO turns a computer into an environment where a child can play, draw pictures, build pictures of pictures, and experiment without being right or wrong. The language makes heavy use of "turtle graphics," a method of drawing figures by specifying direction and distance. For example,

```
forward 10
right 90
forward 10
right 90
forward 10
right 90
forward 10
right 90
```

draws a square. But this can be simplified to:

```
repeat 4
  forward 10
  right 90
end
```

A child can begin using LOGO just like a crayon and paper, and then can save drawings, move them around the screen, scale them, and combine them. In drawing a square, and then giving it a name and manipulating it by name, LOGO provides a simple means for abstraction.

LOGO interpreters are available for the Apple, Atari, IBM-PC, and TI 99/4A computers. If you have a computer that a child wants to play games with, you might offer LOGO instead. Or, if you would like to get a taste of what a very powerful computer language can do, try LOGO yourself.

Smalltalk is another language derived from artificial intelligence. Using a custom-designed minicomputer, Alan Kay and his colleagues developed Smalltalk at the Xerox research labs in the mid-1970s. It is a large, powerful system that is not available on current microcomputers. However, many "revolutionary" concepts, including high-resolution graphics with multiple type fonts, mouse pointing, and pull-down menus, which are provided in the Xerox Star executive workstation and the Apple Lisa and Macintosh computers, were first developed with Smalltalk.

Both LOGO and Smalltalk are powerful languages because they provide functions for manipulating more than just numbers and text. With both languages, more general lists of symbols can be manipulated. Smalltalk also introduced the idea of having functions that could act on complex objects. A system that can perform a few operations on many different kinds of objects is a powerful assistant indeed—a kind of Visicalc for ideas.

MUMPS IS A POPULAR TOOL BECAUSE IT SAVES TIME IN DEVELOPING LARGE PROGRAMS THAT WORK WITH TEXT DATA; IT CAN PROCESS YOUR MEDICAL RECORDS OR MANAGE A LIBRARY CATALOG.

MUMPS

LISP, LOGO, and Smalltalk derive their generality from their ability to manipulate lists, lists that can contain anything from numbers to pictures to antibiotics. MUMPS is a language for processing medical records, and is based on manipulating character strings. Most languages that have character-string variables, such as BASIC and PASCAL, treat strings and numbers as distinct types of data. MUMPS thinks of everything in terms of character strings: character strings may represent integers if they consist of numbers, or real numbers if the numbers contain decimal points. For example, in MUMPS you can write

```
A1 S A=" 7 is."
A2 S B=" 21 divided by"
A3 S C=B/A
A4 WRITE B, A, C
D A1
```

and MUMPS will display

```
21 divided by 7 is: 3
```

MUMPS uses character strings because most medical data comes in words, not numbers. And MUMPS matches patterns to extract data embedded in sentences and paragraphs. Commands are available for matching a particular word, like "tetracycline" or "5 cc", or more general word patterns. The string "1N.N1P3A.A1P2N.N" will match a string containing at least one number ("1N" means match one number, ".N" means allow more numbers), followed by a punctuation character ("1P" will match a space, "-", "/", etc.), followed by at least three letters, a punctuation character, and at least two numbers. So "22-May-84" matches, as does "1 February 1894" or "1984,June,32". The pattern-matching function is often used with a partition function, to separate and move parts of strings. For example, "$PIECE("27-Feb-1984","-",1)" returns "27".

In addition to its string-manipulation commands, MUMPS also provides a database facility. Most database programs are designed to build and manipulate files of fixed-length records. That is, when the database is first defined, each record of information is a certain size, perhaps 80 characters, and each piece of information in a record is at a specific location. For example, a pharmacist's database for his inventory might include a 30-character drug name, a 5-letter abbreviation of the manufacturer's name, etc. MUMPS can build tables of information of any length, so that data on patients with different histories can be stored and searched. MUMPS uses a sophisticated storage technique called "B-trees," which allows information to be added, scanned, and deleted very efficiently.

MUMPS stands for the *M*assachusetts General Hospital *U*tility *M*ulti-*P*rogramming *S*ystem, and most minicomputers running MUMPS also use a MUMPS operating system to provide time-sharing services. MUMPS as an operating system has a number of handy commands for interactive data capture. It can easily ask a question and then wait a specific period of time for an answer, but then continue the program if no response is forthcoming. This, together with treating all data as character strings, makes it easy to write interactive programs that do not get upset when the words "seven" and "yesterday" are typed instead of "7" and "May 19".

MUMPS is a popular language because it saves time in the development of large programs that work with text data. In addition to processing medical records, MUMPS is used in many libraries for storing and retrieving author/title catalog information. But MUMPS is more of a super-BASIC than a PASCAL. Most commands in MUMPS are abbreviated as single letters, and the GOTO (G) statement is used heavily, so programs can be very hard to read and understand. MUMPS is implemented as an interpreter, and it can be very slow, especially for large data-processing problems. MUMPS has little difficulty keeping up with a person typing information from a keyboard, but manipulating thousands of records from magnetic tape can be much more taxing.

In the past two years, versions of MUMPS have become available for microcomputers. MicroMUMPS can be used on CP/M-based 8080 and Z-80 computers, and another version is now available for the IBM-PC. These programs run under the computer's normal operating system, but programs and data are stored in large disk files that can be read only by MUMPS. The programs are available for a modest copying charge, currently $56. If you are thinking about organizing a card file of bibliographic references (or even recipes), you should consider MUMPS.

NONPROCEDURAL LANGUAGES

All the languages we have discussed so far can be used for writing computer programs. However, it is possible to "program" without learning a computer language. Developing a spreadsheet with a program like Lotus 1-2-3 is "programming" of a very easy kind. Spreadsheet programs also provide a key substitution or MACRO facility, which allows text substitution.

It is possible to write programs in 1-2-3 by assigning a string of 1-2-3 commands to a particular key or variable name, and then calling up the variable or pressing the key. Some text editors have an even simpler programming capability; you can press a key and start recording your keystrokes, and then press a second key to repeat the series of commands. This can make it much easier to replace or move blocks of text repeatedly.

The retrieval languages with the popular database programs, such as dBASEII, are also examples of nonprocedural languages. With dBASEII, you first design a database by specifying the size of the fields that will make up the records and the kinds of data to be stored, and then retrieve data by answering a few questions. (dBASEII also has a more conventional procedural language.) This program derives much of its popularity from the fact that the user, not the manufacturer, gets to decide how the database will be manipulated and displayed.

CHOOSING A PROGRAMMING LANGUAGE OR COMPILER

So which programming language should you use? As when choosing a computer, the answer depends on what you want to do. If you just want to learn something about traditional programming, without anything specific in mind, BASIC is certainly the first choice because it is easy to learn, easy to use, and available on most computers. In addition, BASIC will allow you to use many of the machine-specific features of your computer. For example, on an IBM-PC or compatible machine, BASIC is the simplest way to use the graphics and music capabilities.

But be careful. Most hobbyist programmers discover so much with their first programming language that they can't imagine that another language could offer anything more. It is true that almost any computer language can be used to solve almost any problem, but standard Microsoft BASIC is not the best language for many problems. If you are looking for a more advanced language to learn, I recommend Turbo-Pascal for 8- and 16-bit computers, and BDS C for CP/M systems.

You may also need to purchase a compiler because you are converting a program from a mainframe or minicomputer to your micro. If the program is written in BASIC, the transition will probably go well, because the microcomputer BASIC's are very good. (But BASIC programs from some machines with powerful extensions, such as matrix arithmetic, will be more difficult to convert.) If you need to convert a FORTRAN or PASCAL program, several excellent microcomputer compilers are available, but they have limitations. The biggest problem is memory: 8-bit CP/M-based microcomputers must fit the program as well as the data and operating system into 64,000 bytes. A reasonably sized FORTRAN or PASCAL program might require 32,000 bytes of storage, leaving room for less than 8000 4-byte floating-point numbers. This is less of a problem for the newer 16-bit IBM-PC-type computers. The IBM-PC, and the more powerful 68000-based UNIX workstations, should handle minicomputer programs with ease, and mainframe programs with a little work.

Many minicomputer and some mainframe computers build enormous FORTRAN programs using overlays, a technique for sharing a single area of memory among many different subroutines (much like time-shared condominiums). Facilities for using overlays are absent from most microcomputer languages (Digital Research's PL/I is a notable exception). In general, if you are converting a program from a larger machine to a micro, you should try to use the same language, or a more sophisticated language. Converting a mainframe PASCAL program to BASIC would be much more difficult than converting a BASIC program to PASCAL.

The Microsoft FORTRAN compilers for 8-bit and 16-bit computers are excellent. The 16-bit version allows the use of very large blocks of memory, and can use the 8087 floating-point chip to speed up mathematical calculations five- to fifty-fold. The IBM FORTRAN Compiler version 1 (written by Microsoft) was error-ridden, but most of the errors have been corrected in the current version (version 3).

FOR CALCULATION, OR STORAGE AND RETRIEVAL, A SPREADHSEET PROGRAM OR DATABASE PROGRAM WILL PROVIDE YOU WITH ANSWERS MUCH FASTER THAN A GENERAL LANGUAGE LIKE PASCAL OR C.

As I mentioned in the preceding article in this series, Digital Research's PASCAL MT+ for CP/M-based computers, Apple PASCAL, and Microsoft PASCAL (for MS-DOS) are all excellent. These all use UCSD PASCAL extensions to provide subroutine libraries. PASCAL MT+ also has provision for overlaid programs, while the Microsoft PASCAL compiler allows you to play tricks to use large amounts of memory. (Be aware that the tricks allowing the use of large memory blocks subvert much of PASCAL's error checking, though this trade-off may be necessary to fit a large program onto a micro.) Microsoft PASCAL also provides substantial run-time error checking—checks to make certain that array indices are within the proper bounds and that memory is available for subroutine calls. These checks provide a substantial margin of safety for a price; programs sometimes run five times slower with the error-checking feature turned on.

You may also be considering a programming language because there is something that you need to calculate, or store and retrieve, and you are tired of using paper and pencil and index cards. If you are more interested in answers than in computers, it is likely that a spreadsheet program like 1-2-3 or Visicalc, or a database program like dBASEII, will provide an answer much more quickly than a more general language like PASCAL or C. For example, it might take several days to write a BASIC program to collect and plot data from a cell sorter or a gamma counter; and every time you wanted to recalculate or replot, you would have to modify the program. You could probably produce the same results in minutes to hours with a spreadsheet program like 1-2-3 or Visicalc. And the spreadsheet program would be more versatile, making it easy to recalculate and plot different combinations of variables.

Finally, if you don't know anything about computers or programming, but are curious about what these machines can do, remember to try LOGO. It's fun. □

BIBLIOGRAPHY

Most books on languages like C, FORTRAN, and PASCAL can help you with practically any version of the language, because those languages are so standardized. This is not the case with many of the other languages. For example, APL uses a special character set not found on many keyboards. The hardest part of using a microcomputer APL may be figuring out which key means what. For these languages, it might be better to look for books about your specific implementation, and then, after you have learned as much as you can, go on to more general texts. While it is possible to learn about standard programming languages like C and BASIC and PASCAL by reading about them, it is virtually impossible to get a feel for FORTH or LISP or MUMPS without actually sitting down and using them.

FORTH

If you are interested in FORTH, you should write the FORTH Interest Group (FIG), P.O. Box 1105, San Carlos, CA 94070. They sell a number of books on the language. ***The CalTech FORTH Manual,*** Caltech Bookstore, Pasadena, CA 91125 is an inexpensive introduction ($6.50). In addition, the August 1980 ***Byte*** magazine was devoted to FORTH. ***Starting FORTH,*** by Leo Brodie, is available in many bookstores.

LISP

To learn LISP, you will need access to a LISP interpreter. There are two popular versions of LISP in the artificial intelligence community, MACLisp from M.I.T. and INTERLISP from Stanford and Xerox PARC. The two are sufficiently different that you should consider getting a textbook for the flavor of LISP that is accessible for you. ***LISP*** by Patrick Winston and Berthold Horn (Addison-Wesley, 1981) is now a standard text and uses MACLisp. If you just want to learn what you can do with an artificial intelligence language like LISP, consider ***Artificial Intelligence*** by Patrick Winston (Addison-Wesley, 1977).

LOGO

There are several books on how to use LOGO on the Apple, the TI 99/4A, etc. The best book about LOGO describes the philosophy about learning that is behind the language: ***Mindstorms*** by Seymour Papert (Basic Books, 1980). I recommend this book to anyone who wonders whether computers will ever be useful for anything more than balancing a checkbook.

MUMPS

MUMPS texts are very diverse, perhaps because MUMPS is an unusual language with a diverse group of programmers. Two good but very introductory books are ***Introduction to DSM-11*** [DSM stands for Digital Standard Mumps] (1978), which is Digital Equipment Corp order #AA-5457A-TC, and ***Introduction to Standard Mumps*** by Joan Zimmerman (1979), available from the MUMPS Users Group, P.O. Box 37247, Washington DC 20015. MicroMUMPS is available from Dr. Richard Walters, Division of Computer Science, University of California at Davis, Davis, CA 95616.

If you would like to take a quick look at a large number of languages running the same program, look up "Eratosthenes Revisited: Once More Through the Sieve" by Jim and Gary Gilbreath, ***Byte,*** January 1983, pp. 283–326. They compare the results from BASIC, C, PASCAL, FORTH, and many other languages when running a simple program to calculate prime numbers. A sample program listing is presented for each language.

LOCAL AREA NETWORKS: WHY? WHAT? WHAT IF?

DONALD W. SIMBORG, M.D.

The most rapidly developing phenomenon in computing, other than the microcomputer itself, is the technology that links computers. Under the general rubric of local area network (LAN) technology, a new industry has emerged, providing an extensive and confusing array of concepts, configurations, and jargon. Those computing physicians who are still struggling to understand why they require 16 bits rather than 8 are now faced with the decision of using "datagrams" or "virtual circuits" to talk to one of their colleague's computers. Although the technology is complex, the user need only understand it to the level required for making intelligent decisions. This discussion is directed to that purpose.

DONALD W. SIMBORG, M.D.
Dr. Simborg is president of the Simborg Systems Corporation, a company providing consultation and software products for the use of local area networks in hospitals and other health settings. As director of the Hospital Information Systems Department at the University of California (San Francisco) Hospitals from 1976 to 1984, he pioneered the use of local area networks in such environments. He has published widely on many aspects of hospital information systems, and has maintained a practice in internal medicine for seventeen years.

WHY?

Since a network is basically just a connection of multiple computers, why is there suddenly so much interest in this subject? One answer is that since the microelectronics explosion, there are many more computers to connect. But if we are now developing an entirely new and complicated technology to connect computers, why not go back to one big computer again and save the trouble? Why connect one hundred $1,000 computers when I can buy one $100,000 computer?

The simple answer is that 100 microcomputers are more powerful than one larger system costing the same amount, even considering the connection costs. The distribution of computer processing cycles to each user is a powerful phenomenon. It enables rapid response time; it provides independence; and it allows the ultimate flexibility in developing complex information systems.

What's In It for the Computing Physician?

There are many situations in which the computing physician

may use or need a LAN. The most common example is the physician owner of a personal computer which was purchased for use in private practice, in research, or even at home. Suppose, for example, that a number of physicians practicing in the same medical building each own a personal computer for patient billing, basic record-keeping, patient scheduling, or some other functions. Suppose that several decide to keep an expanded clinical database of their patients on their computers, requiring additional disk storage and specialized software.

Rather than each of them investing in this additional expense and effort, they could agree to purchase a single large disk drive and the database software for a new microcomputer, which could be accessed by each of their personal computers through a LAN. In this way they would retain the independent use of their own computers but, through sharing, could take advantage of an elaborate or expensive resource available on another computer.

The clinical databases kept on the large disk can be maintained independently for each of them or, if the same patients are seen by multiple physicians, could be shared for those patients. This saves in hardware and software costs, as well as the time required for each additional physician to enter the same patient information. The LAN could be used for many other purposes, such as sharing other specialized software or communicating via electronic mail. The number and variety of microcomputer networks of this type are increasing rapidly.

The Hospital

LANs are also emerging in quite a different setting. The hospital is an ideal environment to benefit from the power of a LAN. It has an extremely diverse set of functions which could benefit from the use of computers. At the same time, there is a need for communication among these functions because they deal with the same patients. At the University of California San Francisco (UCSF) Hospital, different computers serve the Finance Department, the Admitting and Registration Office, the Nursing Units (for results reporting), the Clinical Laboratory Department, the Radiology Department, and the Outpatient Pharmacy. Those computers were purchased at different times and represent a variety of commercial vendors, hardware, operating systems, and software concepts, yet these systems function as an integrated hospital system as the result of a LAN.

At the UCSF Hospital, the Clinical Laboratory, for example, can purchase the system of its choice in one year, and the Radiology Department can purchase the system that best fits its needs at a different time without constraint with regard to the hardware or software vendor. The hospital system as a whole can evolve in small, incremental steps. Contrast this to the more typical situation in which a hospital administration labors through a time-consuming, costly, and sometimes divisive process of purchasing one large central system from a single vendor—a system which attempts to do everything and winds up pleasing few.

How Many Ways Can You Slice Neapolitan Ice Cream?

There are other settings in which the physician may need a LAN. Suppose the physician is responsible for an organizational unit which already has a large computer serving many users. The use of this computer often grows to exceed its capacity, and response time deteriorates. The combination of the small, powerful computer and the LAN now provides alternatives. These alternatives are analogous to the ways one can slice Neapolitan ice cream. Normally, one would slice the ice cream so that each recipient would have a little bit of the strawberry, vanilla, and chocolate in his slice. Similarly, one way to divide a computer system into smaller computers is to distribute a portion of each of the functions into each computer. Suppose we have a hospital clinical laboratory department computer which performs all of the computing functions for the chemistry lab, microbiology lab, hematology lab, and blood bank. One way to divide these processes among multiple computers would be to have one computer serve the microbiology lab, another serve the chemistry lab, and so on. Although each of these computers would be "dedicated" to a narrower function than the large computer, they would overlap in the types of functions they perform. For instance, each one would maintain its own database of patients, provide mechanisms for input from terminals and for printing of reports, and provide access for the display of results. This configuration allows independence of functions, rapid response time, less vulnerability to CPU failure, and the freedom to acquire modules at different times or from different vendors. Communication through a LAN would be needed in this situation so that the same information about the same patients would not have to be entered redundantly in each of the various subsystems, and a physician on the nursing unit would be able to obtain information from each of the databases through a single terminal.

Consider, however, slicing the Neapolitan ice cream so that one person gets only the vanilla, another only the strawberry, and a third only the chocolate. Although not very interesting for ice cream eaters, it is analogous to another way that microcomputers and LANs are used to divide complex functions. In the clinical laboratory example, suppose that one computer was responsible for maintaining the patient database for all the laboratory sections on a large disk drive; another was responsible for handling all the CRT

COMMUNICATIONS MEDIA

Table 1
Twisted pair wire
Ribbon (flat) cable
Coaxial cable
Fiberoptics
Air (light or radio frequency)

terminals for input and output display; another computer handled instruments, and another computer controlled the hardcopy printers. These various computers are often called "servers" (as in *database server* or *printer server*). Dividing the functions in this manner provides rapid user response time and is efficient in managing shared resources, such as disks and printers. Obviously, the computers in such a configuration are of less value on their own, and are useful primarily because a LAN allows communication to occur among them. Trinity Computing Systems, Inc. markets one such system for cardiology departments.

WHAT IS IT?

Essentially, a network is a connection of two or more electronic devices which are capable of independent control or processing for purposes of data communication. Simply, a network enables computers to communicate. Different kinds of electronic devices, other than computers, are often connected to the networks. These include electronic instruments, imaging devices, or simple terminals which may not be capable of independent processing or control. "Local area" networks should be distinguished from "long-haul" networks. Local area networks are confined to a single geographic location, usually covering only a few kilometers, and function as a single unit with tightly coordinated control of access to the communications channel. Long-haul networks consist of multiple independently functioning systems distributed over virtually unlimited distances. They do not have the timeliness and responsiveness of local area networks. Long-haul networks will not be discussed further in this paper.

The $N^2 - N$ Problem

There has been data communication between computers for decades. Why have there been few LANs until recently? The answer lies in understanding what has been called the $N^2 - N$ problem of computer communications. Consider the example illustrated by Figure 1, in which the objective is to communicate data among three computers, each of a different type. While this may appear simple, the process of passing data from one computer to another turns out to be fairly complicated. Prior to LAN technology, the systems programmers associated with Computer A and Computer B in the example would agree on a communications protocol between the two computers over an agreed-upon physical communications link, such as a twisted pair wire. This protocol could be more or less sophisticated, and would typically deal with such issues as the initial contact mechanism, transmission rate, message length, message delineation, error handling, message flow and sequence, what acknowledgement (if any) the receiving computer would provide to the sending computer, and other issues. Once the specifications for these various communications issues were agreed upon, a computer program was then written for each of the computers to carry them out and allow the communication to occur.

Unfortunately, in most cases the program used by Computer A to communicate with Computer B could not also be used to communicate with Computer C. Since Computer C is different from Computer B, it is likely that there would have to be differences in the detailed specifications of the communications to Computer C, even though it provided many of the same functions. Thus, for the three different types of computers to communicate with each other, there would actually be six computer programs in the network. If a fourth type of computer was added to the network, twelve computer programs would be required to cover all the possible communication links.

Obviously, as more computers were added, using this point-to-point networking technology, the software complexity quickly got out of hand. If N was the number of computer types in the network, then each computer needed N − 1 programs for communication. The

TRADITIONAL COMPUTER NETWORKING

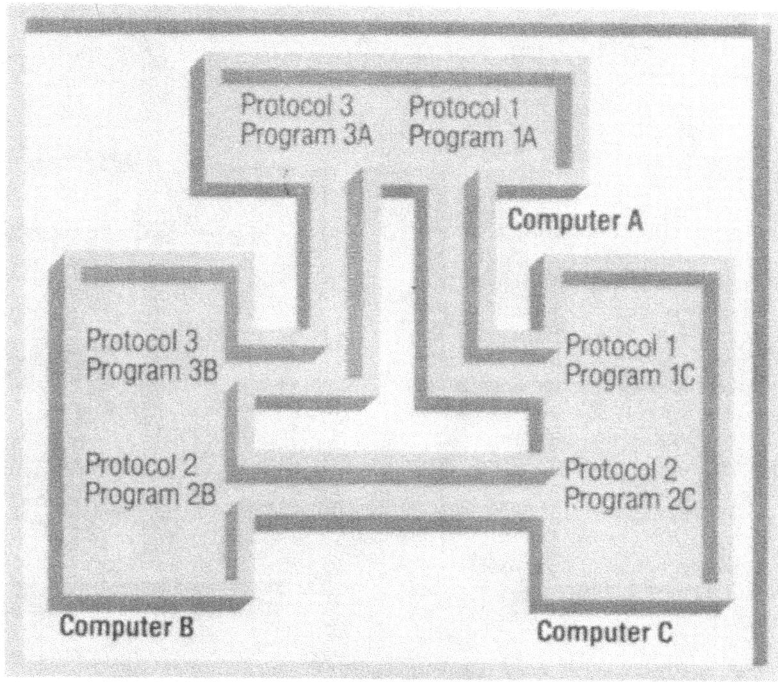

Figure 1

total number of programs in the network was N(N − 1) or $N^2 - N$.

To illustrate the software investment this implies, before the LAN was implemented the development of one such program at UCSF required one year of systems programmer effort. Note also that there had to be many physical wires or cables connecting computers. The formula for this number is $(N^2 - N)/2$.

A decade ago, or even a few years ago, this was not a major issue since most organizations had only one or perhaps two computers. The mini and microcomputer have changed that dramatically. One way to reduce the problem is to require that all of the communicating computers be of the same type or operating system. This simplifies the software, but constrains the options in selecting computers for specific functions.

The Essence of LAN Technology

The essence of LAN technology is to change the $N^2 - N$ problem to an N problem. This is done by removing as many of the communications software functions as possible from each of the communicating computers and placing them in "the network." For the time being, let's consider the network to consist of a series of network devices, as illustrated in Figure 2 within the dark shaded area. The computers talking to the network will be called "host computers." The communications protocol now resides in the network devices which are, in reality, microcomputers, all of the same type. For those communications functions carried out by these network devices, there is only one protocol, regardless of how many host computers there are in the network. Then the problem for each host computer (or other type of host device such as a terminal) becomes one of being able to communicate with its network device—often called a network interface unit (NIU). Once it can do that, it can communicate with any other computer on the network, now or in the future.

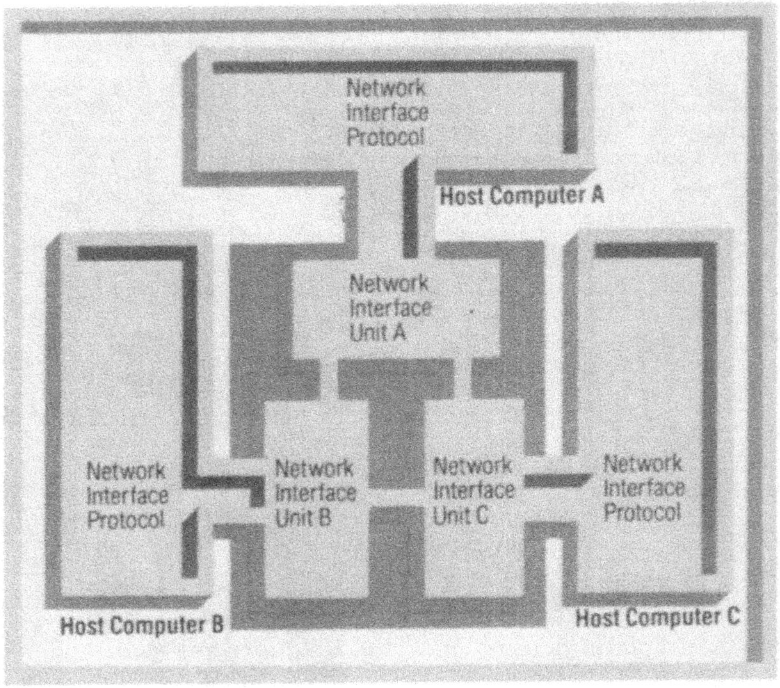

Figure 2

Although the communication between an NIU and its host computer is itself a communications protocol, it is generally less complicated than the protocols illustrated in Figure 1, since many of the functions required for sending data across the network are carried out by the NIUs. The most significant consequence of this configuration is that for each host computer on the network, the only communications protocol necessary is the one required to talk to its NIU. In a network consisting of many types of computers, the number of software programs required to allow communication to occur among all the computers is dramatically reduced. For N different types of computers, there are N communications programs. If all the communicating computers are of the same type, there is only one host computer program, which is replicated throughout all of the host computers.

Understanding The Buzzwords

The network devices shown in Figure 2 consist of network hardware and network software, interconnected by links referred to as the communications media. Media are the physical materials on which the data is communicated between the NIUs (or their equivalents) on the network. Table 1 lists the types of media that are most commonly used in LANs. Generally, the medium is chosen to allow a high data communication capacity in order to accommodate a large number of users sharing the same medium. Typical LANs have a capacity of 1 to 10 megabits (million bits) per second, although higher and lower speed networks are also in use. (At 10 megabits per second, the entire contents of this journal could be transferred in less than one second.) Today, we have the most experience with coaxial cable media, but fiberoptics is becoming increasingly popular. Coaxial cable has the advantage of being easier to "tap" for multiple connections and, at least for the time being, it is cheaper. Its disadvantage is that unlike fiberoptic cable it is subject to various types of electromagnetic noise and interference. Fiberoptic cable is also smaller, lighter, more flexible, and potentially faster for data transfer.

Broadband and Baseband
One commonly hears the terms *broadband* and *baseband* applied to the use of the communications media. In a baseband system, all users of the network communicate by sharing the same communication channel or frequency. This would be like having a single station on your radio. The senders are required to take turns, as the system allows only one communication to be occurring at a given time on the medium. But since the baseband frequency is typically very high, many messages from many users can be interspersed in a relatively short period of time.

In a broadband system, more than one frequency can be used simultaneously, which is like having multiple stations on your radio. The cable can be divided among different sets of users, each using a different frequency or channel. Since broadband technology is the same as that used by cable television (CATV), computer data must be converted to the appropriate analog radio-frequency signal for transmission, and demodulated at the receiving end for conversion back to digital form. This system enables the simultaneous use of a network for many purposes. For example, in a hospital it could be used for computer data, television, voice paging systems, and digital images. There could be more than one data channel, each of which could be considered functionally equivalent to a single baseband LAN. Wangnet, developed by Wang Corporation, is an example of a LAN designed for a broadband environment.

While the broadband system is an attractive idea, the installation of a broadband cable is much more difficult and expensive than a baseband cable because of the special engineering requirements. Technical problems and interference among the various channel users are frequent. More significantly, the degree of coordination and planning among various organizational units has to be much greater. For these reasons, many organizations have chosen to isolate data communications on a base-band LAN from other functions that might share a broadband system.

INTERNATIONAL STANDARDS ORGANIZATION REFERENCE MODEL

Table 2

LAYER	FUNCTION
Physical	Establishes physical connection, and electrical or other representation of bits.
Data Link	Establishes data units, error detection, flow control, access methods.
Network	Establishes information units or packets; provides routing, internetworking (bridges between networks).
Transport	Supports "end-to-end" connection, acknowledgement, virtual circuits, datagrams.
Session	Establishes connection to another host process, monitors communication, manages multiple-message relationships, communicates to user programs.
Presentation	Insures correct data representation and transformation, code conversions, encryption.
Application	Provides dialog with user; interprets, "understands," and processes data; maintains files.

It is likely that very high capacity baseband systems of the future will be able to accommodate voice and television communication in digital form on the same baseband cable used for data. Also, the newer telephone switching systems known as digital PBXs are capable of handling data communications with the telephone service.

Network Topology
The communications medium connects the hardware devices (usually network interface units) which serve the various host computers or terminals that are communicating through the LAN. The configuration or "shape" of the connections among NIUs varies. This is called the network topology. The most common topologies are the ring, star, and bus.

In a star, all nodes connect to a single central point, through which communication passes en route to any other node. A telephone digital PBX is typically implemented in a star topology. Though digital PBXs can be considered as LANs, they are relatively expensive and not commonly accessible at this time.

In a ring, each node or NIU receives messages from its adjacent node and passes messages to the next adjacent node in a single direction around a logical or physical circle. As a message passes around the circle from node to node, each NIU checks to see if the message is addressed to its host. If so, it takes the message off the network. If not, it passes it on.

In a bus network, all nodes are connected to a common communications medium; a message from any one node is heard directly by all other nodes. Each NIU "hears" the message and, if that message is addressed to its host, accepts it. Otherwise the NIU ignores it. Bus networks are becoming the preferred topology because they are less subject to a single point of failure and offer the advantage of the least complicated "broadcast" communications. A broadcast is the transmission of a single message from one node to all other nodes.

Access Methods

In a network in which all NIUs are sharing the same communications medium, there must be some mechanism to allow any particular node to gain access to the medium without interfering with some other node trying to gain access at the same time; otherwise the two signals would be merged on the medium and become garbled. This sort of problem is called a collision. It would be similar to two people speaking at the same time during a conference telephone call.

Two common mechanisms deal with this problem. The first is called contention access. In one type of contention access method, each NIU has two connections to the medium: one for receiving data, or "listening," and the other for sending data, or "talking." When an NIU has a message that it wishes to send, it first listens to determine whether anyone else is using the medium. If not, it begins to transmit its message. It continues to listen while it is sending, however, and for a short period after it is finished sending, to insure that some other NIU did not, by chance, begin transmitting at approximately the same time. The length of time it needs to listen after sending a message depends on the length of the network "cable:" it must listen until a competing message from the farthest node has had time to arrive. This is one major reason for the distance limitation for LANs: the time it takes a signal to travel to the farthest node must be accommodated by the access method.

If it does hear a signal from another node within the appropriate time interval, or detects a garbled message, the NIU knows that a collision has occurred; likewise, the competing NIU has detected the same event. Both NIUs abort their transmissions and wait for a brief interval, randomly determined in each NIU, before beginning to retransmit the same message. It is not dissimilar to what people do subconsciously in conference telephone calls. This type of contention mechanism is often described as carrier sense multiple access/collision detection (CSMA/CD). Ethernet, which is the LAN technology developed originally by Xerox with later collaboration by DEC and Intel corporations, uses a contention access scheme. Ungermann-Bass's Net/One uses Ethernet as the contention access method.

IN A NETWORK CONSISTING OF MANY TYPES OF COMPUTERS, THE NUMBER OF SOFTWARE PROGRAMS REQUIRED TO ALLOW COMMUNICATION AMONG ALL THE COMPUTERS IS DRAMATICALLY REDUCED.

An alternative to contention access is a token-passing scheme. A token is an electronic signal passed from node to node in a ring or bus network. It tells the receiving mode that the medium is available to it for a transmission if required. If the NIU has no data to transmit, it passes the token on to the next NIU. The time allocations for use of the network do not have to be equally shared among all nodes. This can be accomplished by passing the token more frequently to a particular high priority node, rather than always passing it in sequence to every node in the network. Datapoint's Arcnet uses a token-passing scheme.

Token networks have the advantage of insuring a fair or appropriate allocation of the network among the nodes. At very high use of a network, token schemes are more efficient than contention schemes, which are subject to high collision rates. Not only do collisions retard the transmission of the colliding messages, but the retransmissions further increase the use of an already busy network. Token schemes have the disadvantage of being subject to failure through the malfunction of a single NIU, which may "lose" the token or create additional tokens. Also, when usage rates are low, they retard the use of the network by an NIU ready to communicate, which must wait until the token is passed to it. The current debate between proponents of each scheme is not likely to be resolved soon.

WHAT'S IN AN NIU?

The most important thing in an NIU is the network software. Before describing the software, a brief discussion of the hardware is needed. This usually consists of one or more microprocessors, memory boards for storing messages and other functions, and some type of transceiver device for physically relating to the signal required on the medium (which may be digital or analog electronic, light, or radio-frequency waves through air). Often there are two microprocessors sharing memory and other components: one dealing with the host side and the other dealing with the network side of the NIU.

The software must deal with communication with the host *and* communication with the network. The host communication software may vary from NIU to NIU on a single network, since the host computers may vary. Depending upon the network used, this link may be easily adapted to a particular host computer. In other cases, significant programming may be required to adapt the host computer to the NIU. The link between host computer and NIU is typically quite different from that between the NIUs. The host/NIU link may be any one of a variety of typical interfaces to host computers: RS232 asynchronous communication, bisynchronous communication, high-speed serial links, or a special parallel interface. These links have the same spectrum of possibilities as those of any other devices connected to computers, such as terminals, instruments, etc. In the future, NIUs are likely to become an integral part of host computer systems. The visible link between NIU and computer will

WAYS IN WHICH NETWORKS DIFFER

TOPOLOGY	DESCRIPTION	ADVANTAGES	DISADVANTAGES
Star	All nodes connect to central processor.	Simple, no routing decisions.	Failure of central processor causes whole network to fail.
Ring	Nodes are connected in sequence in ring configuration.	Simplicity, predictable message delay.	Failure of one node can disrupt entire network.
Bus	All nodes are connected to a common medium and receive all messages.	Reliable; single failure does not disrupt network. Easy broadcasting.	Contention for bus can slow traffic.
SINGLE VS. MULTICHANNEL			
Broadband	Multiple parallel communications can share medium using different frequency channels. Can mix voice, data, television. Analog signal.	Flexibility. Single medium for all uses. High transmission rates over longer distances.	Complex; more expensive startup; possibility of interference between channels. As yet, little standardization.
Baseband	One communications channel is divided among users in time. Digital signal.	Simpler and more reliable than broadband. Well standardized.	One medium cannot be used for all institutional purposes.
NETWORK ACCESS TECHNIQUES			
Token Passing	Electronic token is passed from node to node in a ring or bus to indicate medium availability. Used in Data Point's ARCNET, and in experimental IBM network.	Tight system control, uniform transmission time even when heavily loaded.	Failure in one node can disrupt the system. More complex to add or remove a node.
Contention Access (CSMA/CD)	"Carrier sense multiple access collision detection." Node transmits when it detects medium is idle. Example: ETHERNET, supported by Digital Equipment Corp., Intel, and Xerox.	Single node failure has no effect on network's integrity. One can add and remove nodes without disrupting network; easy to broadcast messages. Strong standards.	Inefficient when network is used heavily. Modest limits on distance between nodes.
MEDIA			
Twisted Pair	Two wires twisted (like a telephone wire). Transmission capacity depends on quality of wire and distance between nodes.	Low cost.	Limited capacity: 100,000 = bit/sec range. Limited distance.
Coaxial Cable	Used for TV signal transmission by cable TV (similar to round cable connector between VCR and TV set).	When used for baseband, can transmit up to 10 million bits/second; for broadband, nearly 150 million bits/second.	Moderate expense; there can be problems with interface.
Fiberoptics	Light pulses transmitted over glass or plastic.	Lightweight, flexible, immune from electromagnetic interference. Potentially over 1 billion bits/second capicity.	Expensive. Complicated connections.

disappear.

The network-side software is the same in all NIUs of a given LAN. It is here that different NIUs manifest the greatest differences in types of functions and levels of sophistication. Since typically NIUs are physically adjacent to their host computers, transmissions between these two tend to be reliable. By contrast, NIU-to-NIU links can be quite long—thousands of feet. Thus, these links are subject to a high probability of communication errors, noise, etc. It is the software on the network side that determines the reliability and sophistication of the NIU's solution to these problems.

FAILURES CAN OCCUR FOR A VARIETY OF REASONS: NOISY CONNECTIONS, EXTERNAL INTERFERENCE, COLLISIONS, TRAFFIC OVERLOADS, AND HARDWARE OR SOFTWARE FAILURES.

Protocol Layers

Network communications software is commonly described according to a hierarchical model proposed by the International Standards Organization, called the Open Systems Interconnection Reference Model (ISO/OSI). In this model the communications protocol is divided into seven functional layers (see Table 2). In communicating from an application program in one computer to an application program in another, software functions related to all seven layers occur. However, they do not all occur within the NIU. Typically, the lower layers are incorporated in the NIU software, while the higher-level functions are carried out in the host computers. This varies from LAN to LAN; therefore, the degree to which the NIU offloads software from hosts also varies. Some LANs are homogeneous or "closed" systems in which all of the host computers are of the same manufacture or operating system. For such LANs, much of the network software, including sophisticated higher-level communication protocols, can reside in the hosts without paying the penalty of the $N^2 - N$ problem. However, these systems obviously restrict the user's choice to a particular kind of computer or operating system. In addition, such systems may incur a penalty in slower response times because network traffic is competing for the computer's resources.

The ISO model provides an important framework for discussion and standardization among LAN software and hardware designers. But it is confusing to the typical LAN user and, therefore, will not be discussed in detail here.

Network Services

For the purpose of network software discussion it is more useful to consider the types of services and functions that the network software provides to the LAN user. Obviously, all this software must provide some mechanism to communicate on the medium and conform to the access protocol. There are two major services provided by commercially available LANs, however, which tend to distinguish one group of LANs from another. The first is the datagram service, which permits a user to send a discrete single message from one host device to another on the LAN. It is a one-way communication, analogous to dropping a letter in a mailbox. A host device, which could be a terminal or a computer, "drops" messages to its NIU with an appropriate destination address. It can drop multiple messages for the same address, or messages to different addresses. The LAN deals with each message independently to facilitate delivery of each to the appropriate destination NIU, and to the destination host being served by that NIU. Unlike certified mail, there is usually no acknowledgement to the sender that the message was received. Furthermore, there is no guarantee that the messages will arrive in the same sequence as they were sent.

A second important type of service provided by some LANs is the virtual circuit service. This service is analogous to a telephone call between two people. One host device on the network establishes a connection to another host device through their respective NIUs. Once this connection is established, the two end host users communicate directly with one another as though they had a direct two-way connection. The communication is exclusive; i.e., no one else can use the same virtual circuit at that time. As in a phone conversation, the sequence of messages is guaranteed to be the same at the receiving end as it was when it left the sending end. The connection lasts for a variable length of time until it is disconnected by one of the users. Virtual circuits can serve many complex functions, but one common use is to connect a single terminal (attached to an NIU) to a single computer on the LAN. From the user's viewpoint, such a terminal will operate as though it were wired directly to that computer. A few minutes later the terminal could be connected to a different computer through a different virtual circuit. This way, multiple computer systems—say, a lab computer and a pharmacy computer—can be accessed via a single terminal. The Sytek Corporation's LAN software provides a virtual circuit service. Ungermann-Bass Net/One provides a datagram and a virtual circuit service.

Some networks provide another service, the broadcast service. This is similar to the datagram service in that no direct connection is established between end-to-end users. It differs in the number of message receivers. A datagram transmission is one-to-one. A broadcast transmission is one-to-many; that is, to all, or to a subset of the other nodes on the network. In the UCSF Hospital network, we broadcast the patient's new location to all of the ancillary service computers on the network every time a patient is transferred from one ward to another.

Reliability

In evaluating network software it is important to consider not only the type of service, but also the quality of the service provided by the software. Quality depends upon those mechanisms built into the software to insure reliability of transmission and those that attempt to recover from transmission failures. Failures can occur in a network for a variety of reasons, including noisy connections, external interference, collisions, traffic overloads, and hardware or software failures of various types. Some networks provide what is called a "reliable datagram service," as compared to the standard datagram service. In a reliable datagram service, the receiving NIU sends an acknowledgement to the sending NIU when it has successfully received the datagram. It sends a negative acknowledgement when it detects an error in the message transmission. The sending NIU then knows to retransmit the message—which it normally does until it receives a positive acknowledgement or exceeds its re-try limit.

The kinds of error detection and/or error correction techniques employed by a LAN vary. The degree to which host computers are notified of errors on the network also varies. Most datagram services do not provide "guaranteed" delivery of messages between NIUs (in the sense that the LAN attempts to recover from failures or, when this is not possible, to notify the sending host of each failure). In general, broadcast services are even less "reliable" than datagram services in their delivery of messages.

More sophisticated networks provide higher-level services. For example, the 3Com Corporation's Ethernet-based system provides file transfer, file rename, and file delete functions between computers running under the Unix operating system. Discussion of these higher-level services is beyond the scope of this review.

WHAT'S WRONG WITH THEM?

Like any other tool, a LAN can solve a problem only to the extent that the tool is competent and the user is skilled in its use. First, let us consider the competence of the tool. The most important lesson that experienced users have learned about LANs is that they do not totally solve the $N^2 - N$ problem. The NIUs deal only with the lower levels of communication; we still face the $N^2 - N$ problem among host computers at the higher levels. This is a greater problem for "open" networks (consisting of host computers of different types) than for closed systems. It is most apparent at the applications level of communications—the one visible to the physician/user and applications programmer. For example, the clinical laboratory computer may receive patient drug profiles as datagram messages from the pharmacy computer. Successfully receiving data, however, is not enough. The laboratory application program still must be able to interpret that data and use it in application programs such as those that detect drug/lab interaction. The LAN does not understand or care about what is being sent, but only about sending it accurately; yet the application programs do care. If every computer in the hospital network has different conventions about these data (for example, one computer sends a birthdate as Jan. 1, 1965 and another as 1/1/65), the application program in the laboratory computer must deal with these differences individually. Thus, communication is only the first step in systems integration. Now that LANs are available, communication per se does not limit integration. However, application-level incompatibilities still exist.

The problem just described relates to software functions not performed by the network, which must then be dealt with in the host computers. Another consideration is the degree to which the host computers should duplicate functions which *are* provided by the network software. For example, suppose that the network software illustrated in Figure 2 provides a reliable datagram service such that a datagram sent from NIU-A to NIU-B requires a positive acknowledgement to NIU-A of successful receipt of the datagram by NIU-B. Let us further suppose that if NIU-A does not receive this acknowledgement after several attempts, it will notify host computer A of the failure to transmit the datagram. The absence of an error message to host computer A does not necessarily mean, however, that the datagram was successfully transmitted to host computer B.

There are transmission failures that are not recognized by most network software. For example, if an error was introduced in the transmission between NIU-B and host B, NIU-A would never learn about it. Depending upon how likely these types of errors are, and on how important it is for host A to know whether host B received the datagram, the programmers for host A may require the application program in host computer B to send an acknowledgement back to host computer A through the network. This is called an "end-to-end" acknowledgement. The result would be that an error check performed in the network would also be performed at the application level by the host computers. But if the host software duplicates all of the functions of the network software, much of the value of a LAN, i.e., in reducing communication complexity in hosts, is lost. (The value of the LAN would not be totally lost, since error detection and correction at the NIU level would reduce the need for retransmission of messages and implementation of other correction measures at the application level in the host computers.) In reality, a compromise is usually reached. Certain vital functions are duplicated at the "end-to-end" level, whereas others are not. A certain (very low) probability of failure on the network is accepted.

User Skills

Different user skills are required depending on the type of network and how it is used. For a physician who wishes to link his/her personal computer to an existing network, little skill is ordinarily needed. The physician simply purchases the appropriate interface card (equivalent to the NIU) for that personal computer and installs the appropriate hardware connections to the communications medium. The cost may be as low as several hundred dollars, and the software in the personal computer may be as simple as learning to read from and write into a new device. Such a "loose" network is quite adequate for allowing the sharing of a common resource, such as a large disk drive, or for communicating messages through electronic mail.

If the network is going to be used, however, to connect highly independent computer application programs, to maintain shared databases, or to provide an open environment, the skill required of the implementers is much higher. It is a common misconception that a LAN eliminates the need for central control of information systems in an organization. Although it does shift responsibility to the end users to define their own needs for computer applications, it creates an even greater need for skill in the central organization management to insure that, on balance, the needs of the entire organization are met through the integration provided by the network. This relates to the need for network management, monitoring, control software—other variables to consider in LAN planning.

WHAT IF I WANT ONE?

I am often asked the question, "Which LAN do you recommend?" If you skipped ahead to this section, hoping to learn which commercial LAN to buy, you will be disappointed. Those of you who have read the entire article to this point already know that it depends on the answers to many questions regarding the uses *and* the users of the network. There are many kinds of networks, and many uses for them; and there are various levels of resources available to users in purchasing, organizing, designing, and maintaining networks. There is a big difference between a loose configuration of privately owned Apple computers sharing a disk and a tightly interdependent system of heterogeneous computers serving a hospital whose needs are evolving.

When you are considering a LAN, ask the first questions of yourselves—not of the LAN vendor. What do you want to do with the network? What functions will be performed that require data or programs on another computer? How often will that happen? How much data needs to be transferred? How tolerant can you be of errors? After you have thought through your use of the network, then you can determine if there is a vendor product that demonstrably performs similar functions in the hands of another user. If so, how much software development was required to achieve the desired level of functioning?

There is no single technical solution to a given set of functional needs. Datagram services can be used to perform functions for which others use a virtual circuit service, and vice versa. Different topologies, access methods, and media can be used to achieve similar functions. The LAN is only a tool; you must be the carpenter. Whether you plan to rely on a consultant or vendor for assistance in designing your LAN, or are sophisticated (or foolhardy) enough to attempt it yourself, it is my hope that this article will at least help you to ask the right questions and understand the answers. At a time when LAN technology is changing faster than one can pass a token, any answer could be obsolete by the time this issue of *M.D. COMPUTING* goes to press. □

SUGGESTED FURTHER READING

1. Clark D, Pogran K, Reed D. An introduction to local area networks. Proc IEEE 1978; 66:1497.

2. Data processing: open systems interconnection: basic reference model, ISO/TC 97/SC16/N537 (DP7498). American National Standards Institute, New York.

3. Tanenbaum A. Computer networks. Englewood Cliffs, NJ: Prentice-Hall, Inc., 1981.

4. Davis G, ed. The local network handbook. New York: McGraw-Hill Publications Co., 1982.

5. Simborg D, Chadwick M, Whiting-O'Keefe Q, Tolchin S, Kahn S, Bergan E. Local area networks and the hospital. Comp Biomed Res 1983; 16:247.

6. Cotton IW. Local area network tutorial. Los Alamitos, CA: IEEE Computer Society Press, 1984.

TALKING TO COMPUTERS IN ENGLISH

ALAN R. SHAPIRO

Natural languages are those used by people in the course of their daily affairs. This first article deals with so-called *natural language interface systems* (NLIS) which enable users to communicate with computers in ordinary, everyday language, English, for example. Such systems are not science fiction; in fact, several natural language interfaces will be commercially available for use on microcomputers before the end of this year.

WHY NATURAL LANGUAGE?

Familiarity and flexibility are the major advantages of allowing man/machine communication in English. Users with little or no time for learning a programming or query language can still effectively use a computer by using English, a language with which they have personally had years of experience. English has great flexibility for describing concepts (even those we do not yet know how to computerize). However, it is this flexibility and power of expression that makes natural language processing by the computer so difficult.

THE KEY TO NATURAL LANGUAGE PROCESSING: LESS IS MORE

Despite 35 years of research in natural language computer processing, no system to date is capable of intelligent interaction with a human user. Natural language interface systems that have succeeded to any extent have done so either by focusing on a restricted subject, or by using an English language subset small and simple enough to be handled by the computer. This need to focus and restrict will surprise no one who considers the complexity of the communications that ordinary language handles every day. Language must accomodate the complexity and subtlety of a poem by, say, T.S. Eliot, and yet have the clarity and immediacy for a note saying, "Gone fishing."

A request for information stored on a data base management system requires only *a very restricted subset* of the potential sentences that can be formed in English. Yet, until recently, even this restricted domain had been considered too difficult to use as a medium for communicating with computers. As a result, either formal programming languages like Basic, or Pascal or artificially restricted 'English-like' query languages were used. The situation is now changing. The development of a successful natural language interface for medical data bases is promising because the language of medicine itself is a highly restricted, highly structured, and well-defined language.

Ordinary English contains numerous words that have different meanings in different contexts. The sense of these ambiguous words depends on how they are used, i.e., their linguistic environment. Consider words like *vessel*, *film*, *trunk*, *terminal*, *leaflets*, *echoes*, or *regurgitation*. Each has a special meaning in a medical context different from that used in everyday English. Although ambiguous words are not totally absent from medical vocabularies (ROM is an acronym for either "range of motion" or "right otitis media"), they are quite rare. Figures of speech, words with multiple meanings, and the poetic imagery found in everyday English are generally absent. Anatomic words, the names of diseases, drugs, and laboratory tests are usually unambiguous. Therefore, since "medicalese," the argot of medicine, is already a relatively precise and unambiguous subset of ordinary English, the prospect for developing a successful natural language interface to medical data bases appears promising.

QUESTIONS PHYSICIANS ASK OF COMPUTERS

Anyone developing a successful NLIS for medical data bases must study two things first: (a) the clinical vocabulary and the syntax used by physicians and (b) the kinds of queries commonly made by physicians in the clinical setting. To this end, a couple of years ago we performed a simple experiment. We first introduced a group of our residents to a natural language system capable of handling simple requests concerning patient problems and drugs. We then took each resident singly into a room with a "special" computer terminal allegedly connected to an experimental computer system at a well-known institution.

The computer, as we said, could answer any clinical questions residents would care to ask including those about patients in our clinic; and the questions could be put to it in ordinary English sentences. Although the residents were free to ask any category of question in conversational English, their queries were very conventional and characteristic of those handled successfully by the previously demonstrated natural language system, namely, those concerning patient problems and drugs. Such questions as patient compliance, billing, family and other patient characteristics were spontaneously avoided. The experiment seemed to indicate that users accept *structure* in their requests once they know what requests are permitted. For example, the residents could have asked for texts of journal articles or an explanation of why there is sodium retention with congestive heart failure. But they didn't. This implicit willingness to limit the scope of requests is encouraging; it indicates the potential acceptability to users of a limited program for handling a very restricted subset of possible requests.

The terminal, in reality, was not connected to the mainframe at another institution. It was, in fact, connected to a terminal in a nearby room. And at that terminal, like Cyrano de Bergerac speaking unseen under Roxanne's balcony, sat a programmer and a physician, responding to the residents' questions with extraordinary comprehension and eloquence.

Here the residents found a "computer system" that responded appropriately to any query they made. Yet, when asked how useful they thought this system would be to them in practice, 11 out of 15 rated the system likely to be only "moderately helpful" or less.

A full analysis of the results of this "cyranoid" experiment is, of course, beyond the scope of this article; but surely, the experiment suggests that even the perfection of a general purpose natural language interface might not receive the plaudits given to a far simpler specialized interface that was developed for an application perceived as useful in daily practice.

PREREQUISITES FOR A NATURAL LANGUAGE INTERFACE

The most obvious prerequisite for man/machine conversation is the use of a shared vocabulary. Questions then arise concerning whether the shared vocabulary should consist of phrases or individual words. For example, to deal with "mitral valve prolapse" must the system store equivalent phrases, such as "mitral valvular prolapse," "prolapsed mitral valve," "prolapse of the mitral valve?" This approach requires a large vocabulary of equivalent terms and phrases. On the other hand, if the roots "mitral valv——" and "prolaps——" could be stored separately and combined, then the vocabulary could be reduced.

Providing the computer with a knowledge of syntax, the rules by which words are sequenced in English, is a second prerequisite. Interpreting the meaning of questions like "Which patients visiting Dr. Goodman have had hepatitis in the past month?" and distinguishing it from "Which patients visiting Dr. Goodman in the past month have had hepatitis?" clearly depends on a knowledge of which words modify which other words. Syntax has received a great deal of study by computational linguists. However, to process relatively simple retrieval requests, it has been discovered that the computer needs only a minimal knowledge of syntax.

On the other hand, semantics, the meaning of words, plays a major role in many natural language interface systems. Several, such as LIFER (described below), combine syntax and semantics in such a way that the computer can recognize a question like "Which patient had gout?" as an instance of the generic question, "Which patients had ⟨disease⟩?" Any request that begins with "Which patient had______" followed by the name of a disease stored in the system's memory would be recognized by the system and processed appropriately. This approach is called either a "semantic grammar," or, perhaps more accurately, a "pragmatic grammar."

Of course, most conversations between persons are not composed entirely of complete sentences. We frequently resort to the energy-saving tactics of ellipsis and leave out words that are so obvious from the context of our statement that their inclusion is unnecessary. For example, after asking, "Which of Dr. Goodman's patients had mitral valve prolapse?", we might ask, "Gout?" Several systems can handle ellipsis of this sort.

Somewhat more difficult is deciding the words to which a pronoun refers. If the follow-up query had asked, "Tell me those who had gout," the system would need to know that "those" referred to patients in the preceding inquiry. In addition, conventions are needed to define whether "those" refers to all of Dr. Goodman's patients, or instead, only to patients of Dr. Goodman who presented with mitral valve proplapse. Research projects in natural language systems commonly include techniques and conventions for resolving questions of pronoun reference.

A natural language interface system can be susceptible to two types of failures. First, a user may have a particular way of self-expression that the program cannot understand, either because of the user's choice of vocabulary or because of his or her method of phrasing. If the request is reexpressed "correctly," the system can respond. Failures of this type are called failures of *linguistic coverage*.

Requests that the computer program cannot understand no matter how they are rephrased are called failures in *conceptual coverage*. For example, asking a spread sheet program designed for accounting applications, like VisiCalc, to display the "differential diagnosis of hypercalcemia" would result in an inappropriate answer, if not an "error message," no matter how the query was formulated.

CONTEXT: THE MAJOR DIFFICULTY

Most communication depends on assumptions about the background knowledge, perception, and common sense of the person to whom we are talking; the processing of English sentences, as they are literally expressed, are only a small part of everyday conversation. Purely literal interpretation of sentences could have the consequences illustrated in the following hypothetical dialogue between man and machine:

MAN	MACHINE
"Can you tell me which patient had the highest serum uric acid?"	*"Yes"*
"I can't get the natural language interface to understand my question."	*"That is correct."*

MOST COMMUNICATION DEPENDS UPON ASSUMPTIONS ABOUT BACKGROUND KNOWLEDGE, PERCEPTION AND COMMON SENSE...

The first question requests the computer to identify a patient, not to explain the extent of its capability. The second asks for help and doesn't get it. In both cases, the computer misunderstands. In order to make appropriate responses, the computer must recognize the clearly implied intentions of the user.

Although a number of NLIS programmers have attempted to provide a way for the computer to "understand" the contextual nature of a request, a general system with this capability is still beyond the state of the art. Fortunately, requests designed to retrieve information from a data base management system are usually limited enough in their nature so that a computer can be programmed to make "assumptions" about the meaning of the user's requests and respond appropriately.

NATURAL LANGUAGE PROJECTS

1. LIFER (Language Interface Facility with Ellipsis and Recursion)

This system, a product of SRI International in Menlo Park, California, is a rather successful effort that has been adapted to both medical and nonmedical applications. Although its major implementation dealt with answering questions regarding a Naval Command data base, LIFER has been used to develop natural language access to a melanoma data base as well. Examples of questions that the system handles include:

"How many patients are in the melanoma database?"
"How many patients are there with superficial spreading melanoma?"
"How many of them had level 5 disease?"

These queries demonstrate simple retrieval capabilities of the LIFER system. The third query above, although a simple natural language request, requires recognition of pronoun references to the patients identified in the second question. Although simple, several of the systems described below would not have been able to process this request.

The following is another illustrative example handled by LIFER:

"How many patients with superficial spreading melanoma had many mitoses and were followed for 24 months?"

"Many" was previously defined as a value for the variable "mitoses." Other values in the system are "moderate" and "few." However, if a user had asked for "a large number" of mitoses, he would have exceeded the *linguistic coverage* of the system and it would not be able to process his request.

Determining for how long a patient has been followed requires the system to calculate the time between a patient's first and last visits. This ability to handle time relationships between events is unusual in both natural language interfaces and in their underlying database management systems.

"What percentage of these people had histologic recurrences?"

This illustrates the ability of the system to refer to patients found in response to a previous question as well as the ability to calculate averages and percentages.

The LIFER system includes facilities for spelling correction and for defining new terms and asking new questions of the database. For example, if one wished to define a high-risk primary lesion by inputting "Let (HRP1) be defined by (tumor thickness > 1.5 mm and many mitoses)," one could then ask:

"How many individuals with HRP1 were seen for two years?"

LIFER was originally designed for use on mainframe computers. However, it has provided the inspiration for recently developed systems that operate on mini-and microcomputers.

2. SCAMP (System for Conceptual Analysis of Medical Practices)

This system, developed for interrogating a family medicine patient data base, uses a "pragmatic grammar" approach similar to that used in LIFER. Sentences successfully processed include:

"Tell me Dr. Goodman's patients' names with macrocytic anemias who developed avitaminosis and took Allbee with C."

This example shows that the linguistic coverage of the SCAMP system includes the ability to deal with possessive forms and the more subtle capability to distinguish different senses of the preposition "with." The vocabulary of SCAMP has a specific medical orientation. It includes the names of diseases and drugs as well as such "classes" as "macrocytic anemias."

"Which patients developed allergic skin reactions within two months after taking one of the newer NSAIDs?"

SCAMP could process this question because of its ability to handle time relationships among events such as the occurrence of allergic skin reactions and the prescription of nonsteroidal antiinflammatory drugs. The ability to handle such relationships has not been a part of most NLIS even though such relationships can be of great interest, especially in the practice of medicine.

Most systems can process requests for patients who had a certain problem and took a certain drug all in a certain time period, for example, since January 1, 1982. Few systems are capable of handling time *relationships* between events regardless of the date they occurred.

Our experience with SCAMP revealed several problems in using any natural language interface system. First, even the ability to communicate with a computer in English is not a panacea that frees the user from having to learn details about the underlying database. English allows a user great precision in specifying the information for which he or she is searching. However, that precision will be to no avail if the data stored in the underlying database has been collected in a nonspecific form. For example, initially, the medical problems that SCAMP was programmed to recognize were those coded according to the International Classification of Health Problems in Primary Care (ICHPPC), an adaptation of the ICD-9 disease coding system. As a result, queries such as "Who developed mitral valve prolapse?" could not be processed by the original SCAMP system since in ICHPPC this common problem is usually coded under the generic rubric of "All other heart diseases." Users would need to know such details about the data in order to avoid the frustration of a mismatch between the precision of their retrieval language and that of the data.

Another problem noted while using SCAMP is a result of the narrow conceptual coverage of the system. Physicians, when prompted by the CRT screen to "Please enter your request," might type "Which of my patients are candidates for coronary bypass surgery?" And since the system was originally designed to answer only questions about problems, drugs, and the time relationships between the problems and drug-related events, this query would result in a polite but frustrating message "I'm sorry but I don't understand. Could you please rephrase your request?"

The difficulty illustrated here is that when we are invited to communicate with a computer in ordinary language, we tend to think of the computer in anthropomorphic terms. We forget that the machine is likely to have inexplicable and unreasonable gaps in its conceptual and linguistic coverage, making it rather unfit for intelligent discussion. How is it that a machine that knows all the names, dosages, and toxicities of all the nonsteroidal antiinflammatory drugs does not even know the word "candidates"?

We reluctantly concluded that until a *very* comprehensive medical information system was completed, our users need more guidance than is provided by a prompt of "Please type in your request." We turned instead to a menu system in which users are given the freedom to "fill in the blanks" and yet are given guidance about the kinds of requests that can be asked. A similar conclusion, implemented in a slightly different way, was used in developing the Texas Instruments (TI) natural language interface described below.

LITTLE STUDY HAS BEEN DEVOTED TO THE PARTICULAR TASK OF DEVELOPING A NATURAL LANGUAGE SYSTEM FOR MEDICAL APPLICATIONS.

3. INTELLECT

This program was the first commercially successful natural language interface for database retrieval. Originally developed at Dartmouth, where it was called Robot, the Intellect system is now being marketed directly by the Artificial Intelligence Corporation, Waltham, Massachusetts, and, through license, by a number of other firms. The major strengths of the system lie in its adaptability to new databases, referred to as "portability," and in its ability to select possible meanings of ambiguous terms. The creators of Intellect have added graphics capabilities that respond to requests like:

"Show me pie charts for total sales by region for this year and last."

In addition, Intellect can process such requests as:

"List the ages of all patients with gout."
"How many of them took allopurinol?"
"Show their dates of birth."

These last two requests show the advanced capability of the Intellect system in dealing with pronouns, a capability that, like ellipsis, frees the user from much extra typing. One disadvantage of Intellect is that one must be very familiar with the system in order to adapt it to a new database. Reportedly, it takes one week to tailor the system to a new application. Clearly, further improvements in "portability" are needed before Intellect can achieve wide use.

To date, the released versions of Intellect have been expensive, and their marketing has been addressed primarily to large corporations. The above medical examples are hypothetical; we have not seen reported use of Intellect in medical applications although availability of Intellect-like systems for microcomputer users is anticipated soon.

4. SYMANTEC

This company, a spin-off of Machine Intelligence Corporation, located in Sunnyvale, California, has been developing a system intended to be a highly portable natural language interface to data base management (DBMS) systems on microcomputers, specifically, the IBM Personal Computer. At the time of publication, the system had not yet been christened with a name. To minimize problems in interfacing the natural language inquiry capabilities with the data stored on disk, Symantec is incorporating a DBMS as part of its system. The system can process queries like:

"What is the salary of the managers of the older Sunnyvale employees?"
"What is the average salary of the managers of the managers?"

In the second example, the second mention of managers refers to those specified in the first question, a rather impressive demonstration of understanding context. Unfortunately, the system is still under development and its capabilities for practical applications in a medical setting are not yet known.

Symantec is based on LIFER, which you will recall was designed to run on mainframe computers. As a consequence, this adaptation, designed for use on microcomputers, lacks some of the LIFER features. For example, the ellipsis and spelling correction features are missing from the current version of the Symantec NLIS.

Time relationships such as "List the patients who developed gout after January 1, 1982" can be processed whereas time relationship *between* events cannot. Symantec also has graphics capabilities that permit queries such as "Plot the age, salary, and height of female R & D employees."

Announcement of Symantec's debut is expected later this year. Its major advantages are (a) implementation of the program on a microcomputer and (b) ease of use in creating its own personalized natural language interfaces.

5. TEXAS INSTRUMENTS NATURAL LANGUAGE INTERFACE

This system uses a somewhat different approach with its Professional Computer Series. It is based on menu systems for reasons similar to those of SCAMP (see 2 above). Acceptable words that the system can understand are displayed on the screen. After a word is selected by the operator, a list of words that could occur next in the sentence appears on the screen, and again a choice is made. The process continues until a complete sentence is formed. This approach provides explicit guidance to the user concerning the conceptual and linguistic coverage of the system, and it eliminates typing and spelling errors.

TI's natural language interface is designed to process data managed by the Oracle Data Base Management System. Reportedly, some programming sophistication is needed to set up this system for particular applications, although software is being developed to facilitate the process. The system, in its current form, could not handle requests such as:

"Which patients developed jaundice within two months after they took erythromycin estolate?"

without special programming. However, since this question could not be formed from the words on the menu, this limitation would be immediately clear.

At the time of this writing, the TI product has not yet been released, so its convenience, speed, and ease of use in a medical setting remains unknown. The system's designers' experience to date, however, has been encouraging.

NATURAL LANGUAGE INTERFACES VS MENU SYSTEMS

Much research and development has been invested in natural language interfaces. Yet questions remain about the relative advantages and disadvantages of natural language systems compared with menu systems.

A user, told that he or she can communicate with the computer in ordinary English, might well enter such a request as:

"Did any patients with a UTI treated with single dose amoxicillin have two or more recurrences in the following 12 months?"

No current natural language system could handle a request like this without considerable modification. Clearly, the computer would need to choose between the date of definition for the UTI episode or the date of therapy and it would have to know that *recurrences* is a term implying the repetition of a previous event. A true natural language interface would have to be able to negotiate back and forth with the user about the various meanings of the user's requests. Furthermore, without explicit guidance, a user would need to know whether or not data stored in the database was sufficient to distinguish a recurrence from an unresolved course.

On the other hand, menu systems provide immediate guidance to the user and simultaneously reduce the ambiguity of users' requests. Nevertheless, it is also hard to imagine an easy-to-use menu system that could handle the above request adequately.

Little study has been devoted to the particular task of developing a natural language system for medical applications. Until we better understand the capabilities of the systems themselves, the types of requests that physicians would make of such systems, the properties of medical language, the trade-offs between the usefulness of computerized clinical information and the time it takes to obtain it, we shall have difficulty in choosing the ideal approach.

REFERENCES

1. Epstein M: Natural language access to a medical data base. Proc. Second Annual Symposium on Computer Applications in Medical Care, IEEE, 1978.

Applications of LIFER to a medical data base.

2. Hendrix GG and Sacerdoti ED: Natural language processing: the field in perspective. BYTE 1981; Sept: 304-352.

A very good introductory article.

3. Salton G and McGill MJ: *Introduction to Modern Information Retrieval*. McGraw-Hill: New York, 1983, Chapter 7, pp. 257-302.

4. Shapiro AR: The SCAMP system for patient and practice management. J Med Systems 1983; 7:127-136.

A medically-oriented natural language interface and menu system.

5. Tennant H: *Natural Language Processing*. Petrocelli Books: New York, 1981.

A clearly written book on this topic which surveys many of the systems that have been developed.

6. Winogad T: *Language as a Cognitive Process*. Volume One. Addison-Wesley: Reading, Massachusetts, 1983.

Many references; somewhat technical.

ALAN R. SHAPIRO, M.D., M.S.P.H.

Dr. Shapiro has combined the use of computers and quantitative methods in medicine as a systems designer, physician, teacher, administrator and researcher. He has pursued the development of this field while on the faculty of the University of California, San Diego School of Medicine and subsequently at the Stanford University Medical Center before taking on the leadership of a project designed to enhance the availability of medical knowledge to practicing physicians in South Carolina. As Director of the Statewide Family Medicine Computer Network, Dr. Shapiro has developed information retrieval, practice analysis and ambulatory record systems emphasizing the physician-computer interface.

His current research interest focuses on methods for integrating medical knowledge into automated medical records systems. In his free time Dr. Shapiro relaxes at high speed on an ultra-light sailboard of his own design.

The Current State of Operating Systems: 1983 and 1984

PAUL G. TRUAX

Today's office includes many products which did not exist even a short ten years ago. There are intelligent typewriters, personal computers, and multi-station business micros. IBM has just introduced the PC 370, which allows an IBM-XT to run with mainframe software and capability. It has become increasingly important to predict the operating systems that will be most widely used in the future, because the popularity of the one you choose determines the variety, quality, and price of "off-the-shelf" software that will be available to you.

The operating system, without which any computer is just an office sculpture, serves two broad purposes. In the first place, it is the system of control. It manages the priority of the processing, the use of peripherals, the control and progress of tasks being performed; and it provides security and protection for stored information. Secondly, it is the system of application development. It provides the programmer access to programming tools, compilers, and various system utilities. The operating system is also the key to finding existing software.

Various operating systems become popular for different reasons:

1. The operating system may have been made available on a popular manufacturer's product, like the IBM PC (MS-DOS).

2. The system may be extremely easy to use, and therefore attractive to many manufacturers for inclusion with their hardware (the Pick Operating Sytem).

3. The system may have been

PAUL G. TRUAX
Mr. Truax is a well-known information systems consultant, and president of Truax, McElroy & Co. He has authored two books on data collection and systems design, besides writing for the major industry media. He has been quoted by Business Week *and* The Wall Street Journal *on office automation; and has written for* Computerworld, Government Data Systems, The Office, Administrative Management Magazine, *and IBM's Word Processing magazine. He has conducted training programs in Washington, D.C., New York City, Chicago, and San Francisco for McGraw-Hill's Datapro Research Division. He is a regular speaker for the Association of Legal Administrators, the American Management Association, Data Processing Managers Association, International Communications Association, the International Word Processing Association, and many others. He also chaired the Office Automation section of Info for five years.*

extremely powerful for developing certain types of programs such as word processing or math (the Unix [AT&T] operating system).

It is important to identify these winners, since good operating systems will determine the existence and future development of good application software. We must also identify their strengths, weaknesses, and uses. This article will describe the winners and give you an insight into each.

CP/M (CONTROL PROGRAM FOR MICROCOMPUTERS)

CP/M (Control Program for Microcomputers, developed by Digital Research) has been the de facto standard operating system for single-terminal 8-bit computers. However, the great majority of CP/M systems were running on 8-bit CPU chips, either Z-80 or 8080, while 16-bit processors have become standard for stand-alone personal computers. Even though Digital Research developed an outstanding upgrade, a 16-bit product called CP/M-86, the development world had already committed to IBM's MS-DOS, and CP/M moved into a distant second place. Following the tide of users on the IBM PC using MS-DOS, Digital Research converted their library of CP/M-originated languages (CBASIC, PL1) to run under the MS-DOS system.

Digital Research has fought back for its market share by creating CP/M-68 for the Motorola 68000 32/16-bit chip, one of the new generation of supermicrocomputer chips. They also created a version of CP/M-86 which allows for concurrent processing of different computer functions on the IBM PC or its look-alikes. Digital's multi-terminal version of CP/M (MP/M) also fared badly in competition with other products in the 16-bit world. Lacking some of the basic requirements, MP/M had a rough and disappointing startup.

In short, CP/M has been a success only in stand-alone 8-bit systems. Unfortunately, there is little future here. The entire world is moving to 16-bit products, and that includes the home marketplace. Even Commodore, which previously sold only 8-bit computers, has announced a 16-bit home computer based on the ZILOG Z-8000. The real future of CP/M and Digital Research will depend on their ability to provide industry-compatible languages and compilers.

THE REAL FUTURE OF CP/M WILL DEPEND ON THE AVAILABILITY OF INDUSTRY-COMPATIBLE LANGUAGES AND COMPILERS.

MS-DOS

MS-DOS by Microsoft Systems of Washington has become the 16-bit operating system standard for single-user personal computers. IBM uses a proprietary version of this system called PC-DOS, but it is practically the same; applications intended for either will usually run on both. Since 16-bit MS-DOS systems are substantially more powerful than the older 8-bit systems, programs that were written in assembly language for 8-bit systems, like word processing programs, can now be written in higher-level languages, like C.

The use of high-level language makes programmers substantially more productive than if they were writing in an assembly language. Moreover, the software written in C can easily be transported to different computer systems, since C is available in many operating systems. Thus, as technology progresses, software need not be rewritten for new chips and processors. Since IBM is currently installing close to 50,000 personal computers per month, MS-DOS has become a rich field for software development organizations.

The ease of creation and portability of applications written in C, along with the large number of software developers in the field, have created some stiff competition for the dedicated word processor. Most of the original word processing products used 8-bit processors running on totally proprietary operating systems. Their programs, written in assembly language, could take five to eight times longer to write than comparable programs written in higher-level languages like C, RM COBOL, or SMC BASIC. An even greater problem is that assembly language program code is processor-dependent, requiring software to be rewritten as technology changes. Programs are locked into older products.

Multi-terminal requirements in MS-DOS have been met only through networking, which does not yet provide a true multi-terminal, multi-tasking environment. For example, most existing network systems do not permit sharing of files or individual records; and they are costly. However, some of the newer network systems do permit file sharing, and costs will decline. In addition, since MS-DOS is being integrated into other operating systems as a subset system, the multi-terminal requirements will be met in different ways. We see MS-DOS becoming a subset of both Pick and Unix, two excellent multi-terminal, multitasking operating systems.

OASIS 8 AND OASIS 16

The Oasis operating system by Phase I Systems is best known for its multi-terminal capabilities for 8-bit computers. The system is quite powerful because it offers, as an option, an integrated relational database management system called CONTROL.

There is a wealth of languages, file structures, and communications capabilities for Oasis 8. This is by far the best multiterminal 8-bit system available. But Oasis 16 has been slow in coming, and CONTROL is not available on many 16-bit machines. In the 16-bit world, Oasis faces competition from the Unix and Pick systems. Oasis 16 has many of the qualities of Unix (multilanguage and multifile structure) and of Pick (as an integrated database management system). However, these systems had a substantial lead in the market because Phase I was slow in introducing its version, allowing the competition to grow much larger software libraries. Oasis cannot compete in systems larger than 32 terminals, and will not within the near future.'

THE UCSD P SYSTEM

The UCSD P system was created at the University of California at San Diego, and is currently maintained and sold by SofTech MicroSystems. The P system uses an intermediary program code called "P code" to implement the operating system. Thus, it is necessary only to encode the P code functions on a new computer chip or computer system; the operating system is then run as a program written in P code. Thus, it is unusually easy to implement the UCSD P system on a variety of processors. In fact, the system is operational on both 8- and 16-bit units, and is said to be the most processor-independent of all operating systems. It is based on UCSD Pascal, which is its primary language.

The UCSD P system is found on a wide variety of personal computers but on few larger systems. It is not available on supermicrocomputers or minicomputers other than the DEC PDP-11. It has been implemented on the IBM Displaywriter, the IBM PC, and other stand-alone PC products. Most of the multi-terminal versions are implemented as a network of stand-alone PCs, all sharing a hard disk via the network.

The system has not been as well accepted as other systems by general users, but has been well received among scientific and educational organizations. All programs are compiled in the intermediary P code. This approach allows different parts to be written in different languages but compiled in the common P code, providing one integrated program. The mixing of languages makes for an excellent development environment but, because of the compiling procedures, leads to programs that run slower than those written in the traditional compiled languages of other operating systems.

THE PICK SYSTEM

The Pick System, developed by Pick Systems of Irvine, California, has been around for over twenty years, starting as a development project for the United States Army. This product has one of the broader ranges of implementation, from large mainframes down to the IBM PC. Its original market strength did not emerge from the PC market, but grew out of the 16-bit minicomputer and the IBM 360 mainframe. This operating system is both multi-terminal and multitasking, and it uses variable-length records (previously limited to 64,000 characters, but now without limits) in its files. The operating system is implemented on products of many manufacturers, including Digital Equipment Corporation, Microdata, Hewlett Packard, General Automation, IBM, Honeywell, Altos, Data Media, and Pertec. It is used on personal computers, multi-terminal micros, minicomputers, superminicomputers, and mainframes. The implementations are tightly controlled by Pick Systems, and therefore are compatible from brand to brand, and from one product class to another. Thus there is a very large pool of quality software in just about all major markets, including medical practice, distribution, education, finance, and manufacturing.

The system is probably one of the easiest to use because of its integrated database design. In a business environment where large amounts of data are being stored, updated, and retrieved, it is unique. It uses English syntax and sentence structure to manipulate data and files; for this reason, the system is equally useful to the systems analyst and the end user. It has the largest volume of vertical (industry-specific) software in the multi-terminal marketplace.

So far, this system has been especially weak in word processing. However, within the next several months Pick will integrate MS-DOS as a subset. When this occurs, all of the superior software for office automation and word processing found on the IBM PC will become available to the Pick users. Other integration efforts to combine this operating system with Unix and IBM's MVS and VM will make the software from any of these environments available to the users of the others. This will create an incredibly large pool of "generic" software.

In the future I see Pick being implemented on the IBM Mainframe as an application under IBM's MVS, as it already is under VM. This will allow for a new level of programmer efficiency which is not possible in the complex user-unfriendly operating systems. All of the implementations are either 16- or 32-bit, and range from single-terminal systems to 256-terminal systems. These terminals can be either smart or dumb, and can range in price from $500 for one that gets all of its capability from the central processor to $6,000 for a totally compatible PC standalone. Several third-party companies have created a wide range of communications software, including a full range of multi-CPU networking products. When Pick is implemented under MVS or VM in IBM systems, the full power and sophistication of these mainframe central processors and operating systems are available to the user.

UNIX HAS EXCELLENT DEVELOPMENTAL TOOLS, AND MOST MAJOR LANGUAGES ARE AVAILABLE–A SYSTEM DEVELOPER'S DREAM.

THE UNIX SYSTEM*

The Unix system was created by Bell Labs in the mid-1970s. Originally this operating system was implemented internally in the Bell System. Later, it spread rapidly to the college and university marketplace. Its avid fans on college campuses have enhanced the system many times over. Unix is especially strong in text processing and office automation. It has many excellent development tools, and most major programming languages are available—a system developer's dream. Cross-compilers are also available, allowing for

*Unix is a registered trademark of Bell Laboratories.

conversion from one language to another. The system's primary language is C, in which the operating system itself is written.

Programmers especially like this system because it can run many tasks simultaneously. However, end users find the system "unfriendly." For their use a database management system should be added.

As mentioned earlier, Pick may be implemented in the future as the primary relational database application within Unix. This should allow Unix to have the same utility to end users as to software developers, and will surely give both operating systems a broader range of appeal. Both systems are time-tested multi-terminal, multi-tasking operating environments.

Because of its wealth of development tools and variety of languages, I feel that Unix will be found at the base level, with Pick and others being more often implemented as the application. Also, because of its unique capabilities in simultaneous processing Unix is better suited to manage peripherals, interrupts, tasks, and security. Unix is quickly becoming the standard in the 32-bit computer world, especially at the base or controlling level when more than one operating system is present within the same computer system. Hewlett-Packard, for example, has just announced its intention to place Unix as controlling system for all its future mini and mainframe products.

Pick is also a strong operating system, but it is far better suited than Unix to managing large amounts of data, and can be more easily run without the data processing guru. For these reasons, I predict that the inevitable will occur—Pick and Unix will soon be integrated. Until that happens, Unix will be most often found in the hands of the programmer, while Pick will more often be found in business or database management environments.

MUMPS: A SPECIALIZED OPERATING SYSTEM

Most of the operating systems discussed in this tutorial are general-purpose; that is, they are designed to allow the user to apply the computer hardware to many software tasks. These operating systems support many different programming languages, different database and file management facilities, a variety of software tools, etc. The general-purpose nature of these operating systems provides a broad capability, but at a price in performance. There is an alternate philosophy: develop and optimize an operating system for a specific language or environment and optimize the processing. The idea is to obtain performance gain by specializing. The cost of this is loss of the flexibility of a more general operating system.

The MUMPS operating system is an example of an operating system designed for a single language. While the language MUMPS runs under many operating systems, the MUMPS operating system supports only this one language. Naturally, one should expect the best performance when the specialized operating system is used.

MUMPS stands for the Massachusetts General Hospital Utility Multi-Programming System. As both the name and acronym imply, MUMPS had its origins in the medical community. But the use of MUMPS is not limited to medical processing; today, half of its applications are in commercial facilities. Nevertheless, the primary objective in developing the language was to provide a powerful and inexpensive facility for the interactive processing of medical data.

MUMPS was first developed in the late 1960s. When the concept of time-sharing was introduced, interactive computing was just entering the commercial marketplace. But interactive programming was expensive. Alternate solutions were sought, and the new "minicomputers" offered an alternative.

Briefly, the MUMPS operating system was designed to support many interactive users performing database operations on a small computer with limited memory and mass storage—and to do this efficiently. Since the late 1960s, minicomputers have grown to the size of the old mainframes, and a new generation of microcomputers has taken the place of the old minicomputers. The problem is the same: how can one get effective, multi-user, interactive database systems using the limited resources of a microcomputer system? General-purpose operating systems offer one approach; a dedicated operating system is another.

In order to appreciate the MUMPS system, one must know something about the language. The key to MUMPS is its ability to manage strings of characters, such as a name, diagnosis, date, or result. MUMPS has a very simple syntax which makes user interaction very easy. Even more important, it has a powerful database manager which makes storage and retrieval both rapid and efficient. Data are stored in a natural hierarchy; for example, you might request the WBC result for the 12/17/83 visit of the patient Jones. The language allows one to read or write this datum as if it were in a multi-dimensional array. There are no declaration or dimension statements, no job control language, nothing to get between the user and the application.

The function of the MUMPS operating system is twofold: to provide utility programs to save and restore files, etc., and to be invisible to the user while improving throughput. The appeal of this operating system will obviously be limited to those who plan to program all their applications in MUMPS. Users of COSTAR—a MUMPS-based medical record system—represent one such group; there are many others. While it is not suited for applications with a heavy computational requirement, it is ideal for flexible, efficient interactive database systems.

BRUCE BLUM

Unix currently suffers from lack of standardization. There are no less than fifty different versions. Standardization will come as AT&T increases its level of support for the product and begins to sell its own hardware; the other vendors who use Unix will then follow the AT&T standard. This will increase the portability of software and create a larger overall software pool.

VM

VM is the IBM mainframe operating system to watch. This product is migrating rapidly into the supermini, mini, and microcomputer product classes as well. However, when the user company desires to implement a full set of IBM's communications standards such as SNA (Systems Network Architecture) for multi-CPU networking, MVS (another IBM operating system) is necessary as the controlling system. Both VM and MVS systems can support other operating systems running as applications. However, VM is implemented at all levels from micro to mainframe, and is the most hardware-independent.

These operating systems are especially important in organizations with a large inventory of existing applications. Older IBM operating systems can be run as applications under VM. Thus, an organization is free to use new software applications running under VM while continuing to use their existing programs running under an old operating system on the same machine. The generic system of Pick is currently available under VM. This is important, since operating systems like Pick can provide a five-fold to eight-fold productivity improvement over the native mainframe operating environments.

VM has just been announced for the IBM XT PC 370 (an IBM personal computer with a special board in it). This development is valuable to large companies since VM can provide a thread of compatibility to all levels of systems in these organizations. Nevertheless, several key points must be made regarding the significance of this announcement:

1. Mainframe applications can now be run on (or downloaded into and run on) the IBM PC XT 370.
2. Mainframe applications can be developed on the PC XT 370 (but only by mainframe professionals) to be run on the mainframe.
3. End users will still not be able to develop their own applications on these units unless the VM system has a friendly application development shell such as Pick.
4. Though VM is available to the local department or single user via the XT 370, the system is only being offered as a single-user stand-alone. (It is forecast, however, that the XT 370 will become multi-terminal within one year.)
5. IBM is expected to introduce a desk-top version of its 4300 minicomputer which will also run VM, but in a multi-terminal mode.
6. Small businesses would be better served by going to a less complex operating system running in a native mode (not under VM) since they would not require IBM communications. These companies would be well advised to develop applications either in Unix with a friendly interface or in Pick alone. They should concentrate on existing software, since there is a wealth of software for most industries in both Pick and Unix.

In summary, VM exists for three main reasons:

a. VM provides the bridge between the older, more complex IBM operating systems and the newer generic operating systems. It can act as a base/controlling operating system for both the old and the new, thus preserving a library of developed software.

b. VM will in the future provide a base for IBM's main communications plans.

c. VM provides the link to the future since it is hardware-independent, allowing this system to move with technology.

MANY OPERATING SYSTEMS WILL SOON BE AVAILABLE TO EACH OTHER THROUGH CROSS-COMPILERS OR APPLICATION GENERATORS, OR BY HAVING ONE RUN WITHIN ANOTHER AS AN APPLICATION.

CONCLUSIONS

I believe that all computers must become generic; those that resist the evolving de facto standards will ultimately fail. Proprietary operating environments will no longer be tolerated, because the consumer wants (and should demand) the broadest base of application software and the flexibility to change hardware suppliers. In the very near future, many of the operating systems discussed in this report will become available to each other, either through cross-compilers, through application generators, or one running within another as an application. Four of these systems will be dominant in the future:

MS-DOS will remain the standard for all personal computing in a stand-alone processor.

Pick will remain the standard for multi-terminal systems where business and database management applications are predominant. The system should be installed where it is not important to have full-fledged DP professionals on staff, or where the end users may be developing applications. Alternatively, it may be installed as a friendly application shell under Unix, or under an IBM mainframe operating system such as VM.

Unix will remain the standard for the software developer or data processing professional. It will also remain the best system for developers of word- and text-processing applications. It is the best system for the connection of many foreign device attachments.

VM will become the standard in the mainframe environment for multinational corporations where an overall corporate scheme of computers and networking is necessary. However, VM must coexist with higher-level development tools for programmers (meaning Unix) or for programmers and end users (meaning Pick). We feel that VM alone is too complex for a small corporation or services company.

Any one of these systems is a safe haven for the user, since in the future all four operating systems and their associated applications software will be available in many combinations. For now, however, users should select the operating system that is best suited for their needs today. □

AN INTRODUCTION TO LISP

MICHAEL G. WALKER AND ROBERT L. BLUM, M.D., Ph.D.

This article, the first of two tutorials on programming in Lisp, introduces the language and shows you how to program in it. In a future issue we examine a miniature "expert system" called Minimycin. Expert systems are computer applications programs that use artificial intelligence (AI) techniques to perform a task normally done by human experts. We designed Minimycin to show how Lisp can be used to create a rule-based expert system.

WHY LEARN LISP?

Besides being fun, Lisp has been the lingua franca of artificial intelligence research for the past 25 years. One of the oldest high-level programming languages, Lisp was designed in the late '50s by Professor John McCarthy, then at MIT. It is just a few months younger than FORTRAN, the widely-used mathematical processing language. Lisp is the major language used in expert systems, robotics and vision systems, and language translation systems. Its only serious competitor is PROLOG, which is increasingly popular in Japan and Europe but used at only a few research centers in the United States. With several companies (Symbolics, LMI, and Xerox) now manufacturing computers designed to run Lisp exclusively, it is likely that Lisp will continue to be the main AI language for the next decade.

Lisp has several valuable features suited to AI. Their meaning and value will become clearer as you learn more about Lisp and expert systems in these two articles. Briefly, Lisp's advantages for an AI context include:

1. easy symbol manipulation (as opposed to numeric manipulation);
2. complete equivalence of programs and data;
3. many convenient tools for knowledge representation (Lisp stores data as lists of characteristic properties and logical associations; this is more natural to human thinking processes than FORTRAN, for example);
4. a highly interactive programming environment for both users and program builders;
5. built-in tools to find and correct bugs, edit, help correct syntax, and analyze programs.

MICHAEL G. WALKER
Michael Walker is a Lisp programmer in the Computer Science Department of Stanford University, and a systems engineer in Intellicorp's Knowledge Systems Division. He has been involved in projects in artificial intelligence and databases since 1979. He is a member of the American Association for Artificial Intelligence and the ACM Special Interest Group on Artificial Intelligence, and is also a reviewer for IEEE Computer Magazine *and the Conference on Very Large Data Bases.*

ROBERT L. BLUM, M.D., Ph.D.
Dr. Robert Blum graduated from the Massachusetts Institute of Technology in 1969 with a bachelor's degree in mathematics. He received an M.D. from the University of California Medical School at San Francisco in 1973. For the next three years, he had an internship and residency in the Department of Internal Medicine at the Kaiser Foundation Hospital in Oakland, California, where he was Chief Resident in 1976. From 1976 to 1979 he was a Post-Doctoral Fellow in the Stanford University Division of Clinical Pharmacology. He also received a Ph.D. in computer science and biostatistics in 1982 from Stanford University.

Since 1979 Dr. Blum has been the principal investigator of the RADIX Project in the Stanford Computer Science Department. The goal of the RADIX Project is the automated discovery and confirmation of medical knowledge from large clinical databases. This project's interests center on the merger of database technology, statistical methods, computer representation of medical knowledge, and heuristic methods of discovery.

The rest of this article introduces you to the building blocks of the Lisp language: atoms and lists, equivalence of programs and data, values of atoms, predicates, properties of atoms, conditional expressions, the Golden Rule of AI, rule evaluation, and program control through iteration and recursion.

ATOMS AND LISTS

Like the Universe, Lisp is built of "atoms." An atom is a single text "word" consisting of contiguous letters or numbers (and a few other permitted characters) followed by a blank space. Here are six examples of atoms:

```
ALICE  375  PATIENT-532  14.57   (4 atoms)
THIS-IS-A-VERY-VERY-LONG-ATOM
GLOMERULONEPHRITIS,MEMBRANOUS
```

Here are six more examples of atoms:

```
ATOM?   IF      PLUS
PRINT   TIMES   MULTIPLY
```

Some characters—left or right parentheses, for example—cannot be included in atoms, since they serve functions in Lisp's grammar or syntax.

A "list" is a sequence of atoms wrapped in parentheses. Lists are sometimes called "s-expressions" (for *symbolic expressions*) or simply "expressions." We refer to them as expressions when we want to emphasize their dual nature as "little computer programs"—but let's not get ahead of ourselves.

Here are three lists which contain one, two, and five atoms, respectively.

```
(A)
(GROCERY LIST)
(BREAD CHEESE WINE AND THOU)
```

A list may consist of atoms and/or other lists. Each item in a list is called an element (Figure 1).

It is important to balance your parentheses. Be sure that every list has an opening and a closing parenthesis. The Lisp interpreter will complain vigorously when you forget.

This is correct.	(A (B C (D)))
This is not correct.	(A (B C)

LISP HAS BEEN THE LINGUA FRANCA OF ARTIFICIAL INTELLIGENCE RESEARCH FOR THE PAST TWENTY-FIVE YEARS.

You may agree with some people who think "Lisp" stands for Lots of Irritating Single Parentheses. Fortunately, there is one exception to the rule. Lisp allows you to terminate any number of left parentheses by a right square bracket "]". Thus, "(A (B C (D)))" can be written: "(A (B C (D]." This saves lots of typing and usually makes the list easier to read.

Programs Equal Data

Atoms and lists are the only data structures used in Lisp. But recall that in our list of useful features, we noted that in Lisp, programs and data are equivalent. Any Lisp statement can be regarded as a program or as data depending on the context. Look at the following sample programs. Notice that they are lists.

Program	What it does
(PRINT 7)	*Print the number 7.*
(SETQ Z (PLUS 3 4))	*Add 3 to 4, then set Z to have the value of this sum.*
(PRINT Z)	*Print the value of Z (determined to be 7 by the previous program command).*

Lisp programs accomplish things through "functions." In our example, the atoms PRINT, SETQ, and PLUS, are the names of functions that print, set a value, and add, respectively.

Another very important characteristic of Lisp is that every function returns a value. For example, although (PLUS 31 5) adds 31 to 5, it also returns a value, which happens to be 36. So if you write (PLUS 7 (PLUS 31 5)), the first PLUS will add 7 and 36, and will return a value of 43. As the first step in evaluating this expression, the computer converts the expression into (PLUS 7 36). At the next pass it converts the new expression to 43.

This is so important that we'll say it again: *every function in Lisp returns some value.* So (TIMES 7 2) returns 14; (PRINT 7) first prints a 7, and then returns a value of 7. (SETQ Z (PLUS 3 4)) returns a value of 7, and so on. What this means when you are developing a program in Lisp is that the results of a function are immediately available for a new action or evaluation. As we will see later, this allows the program to follow complex strings of branching logic.

FUNCTIONS IN LISP

The following examples are presented as though you were at a computer terminal interacting with Lisp. When Lisp presents the prompt "_" on the screen, you respond by typing in an atom or a symbolic expression (a list). Lisp responds to a valid expression by returning the value of the atom or expression you entered. [User input is underscored throughout this article.] For example:

Computer	User	Comments
_	(PLUS 3 4)	
7		*Lisp shows the number 7 on the screen.*

Lisp evaluated the symbolic expression (PLUS 3 4) and returned the value 7.

We call PLUS, PRINT, SETQ, and so on, *functions*, because like mathematical functions they map the value of one or more arguments to another value. That is, PLUS takes the arguments 3 and 4 and gives back their sum 7.

Functions always have the form:

```
(Function-name Argument-1   Argument-2 . . .
Argument-N).
```

The first atom in the list is the name of the function, and the remaining atoms are the arguments—the things that the function works on. Since arguments are just elements of a list, each one may consist of atoms or lists.

The function (PLUS 2 (PLUS 3 4)) works as follows. This is a list with three elements: PLUS, 2, and (PLUS 3 4). Lisp sees that the first atom is the name of a function and evaluates that function using the two arguments which follow. The value of 2 is just 2. The value of (PLUS 3 4) includes a function, so Lisp applies the function to its arguments, 3 and 4, and returns the value 7. The first PLUS now has a value for its second argument and can complete its work to return 9. (Actually Lisp "reads" from the inside out, finding and evaluating the element with the most parentheses first.)

So far we have only shown Lisp evaluating lists. But atoms can also have values. (In some ways an atom is similar to variables in other computer languages, since it can be assigned values. However, unlike many languages, Lisp does not restrict the values of its "variables" to a specific kind of data, e.g., just numbers.) SETQ assigns values to atoms. So (SETQ X 7) sets the value of the atom X to 7 and also returns the number 7. Try it yourself. If we type: (PLUS 1.5 (SETQ X 3)) at the terminal, what do we get back? The answer is 4.5. The computer has also set the value of X to 3, so if we type X at the terminal Lisp will print 3. (See Figure 2.)

TYPICAL LISTS AND ELEMENTS

Figure 1

EXAMPLE	COMMENTS
(THE HARE WAS LATE)	*A list with four elements, each an atom.*
(CAT (FAT) NAME (GARFIELD))	*Another list with four elements. The first and third are atoms; the second and fourth are also lists.*
((ALICE HATTER) (RABBIT QUEEN))	*A list made up of two elements, each a list with two atoms.*
(PATIENT-1 AGE 32 SEX FEMALE RACE CAUCASIAN CHIEF-COMPLAINT NAUSEA DX PREGNANT)	*A list with eleven elements, each an atom.*
( )	*An empty list—perfectly respectable, but with no elements.*
(A (NESTED (LIST WITH TWO ELEMENTS)))	*A list with two elements. The first is the atom "A". The second is a list "(nested (list with two elements))", one of whose elements is also a list with 4 atoms: "(list with two elements)".*
(RULE4 [IF (AND (PATIENT IS FEMALE) (PATIENT IS AN ADULT) (PATIENT HAS DYSURIA))] [THEN (BACTERIA IS E. COLI)])	*A list with three elements. The first is an atom, "RULE4". The second is a list starting with "IF". The third is the list starting with "THEN".*
((AN (EXAMPLE (OF A) (DEEPLY (EMBEDDED LIST)))))	*This is a list with only one element: a list begining with "AN" and ending with "LIST". The elements within that list are also lists.*

The Values of Atoms

So far, we've only given atoms numeric values like 3 and 4. Atoms can also be given arbitrary values. The value of an atom can be another atom or even a list. Look at the next example.

```
(SETQ CHARACTERS '(ALICE HATTER
   RABBIT QUEEN))
(ALICE HATTER RABBIT QUEEN)
```

On the first line, we set the value of the atom CHARACTERS to be the list (ALICE HATTER RABBIT QUEEN), and Lisp printed out (ALICE HATTER RABBIT QUEEN) on the second line as the value of the SETQ expression. The single quote mark " ' " is used to tell Lisp that we want to set the value of characters to be literally the list (ALICE HATTER RABBIT QUEEN) and not its value. The examples in Figures 3 and 4 illustrate this point.

This process of evaluating an atom or an expression is all that Lisp does. When you type something to Lisp, it evaluates your input, treating the first atom it sees as a function and the succeeding atoms as arguments.

This process of evaluation of atoms and functions can be arbitrarily nested inside Lisp expressions, as we see in Figure 4.

Note this last example in Figure 4 carefully. We called a function named EVAL. EVAL just tries to obtain the value of whatever its argument is. But this is all the Lisp interpreter itself does when we type an expression into the computer after the prompt. The function EVAL allows us to invoke this process anywhere, arbitrarily.

Before we challenge you with some real puzzles, let's enrich your Lisp vocabulary with a few other built-in functions besides PLUS, TIMES, and PRINT.

APPEND glues lists together. So (APPEND '(CHESHIRE-CAT GARFIELD) '(WALRUS CARPENTER)) returns the list (CHESHIRE-CAT GARFIELD WALRUS CARPENTER). This is useful when you want to add a new set of characteristics to a set already in your data bank, or when you want to add new findings to a list of patient findings.

CONS glues an atom to a list. So (CONS 'QUEEN '(TWEEDLEDUM TWEEDLEDEE)) returns the list (QUEEN TWEEDLEDUM TWEEDLEDEE).

LIST wraps parentheses around its arguments. So (LIST 'ALICE 'HATTER) returns the list (ALICE HATTER). (LIST 'CHESHIRE-CAT '(RABBIT) '(HATTER)) returns the list (CHESHIRE-CAT (RABBIT) (HATTER)).

REMOVE takes an atom out of a list. So (REMOVE 'CHESHIRE-CAT '(ALICE CHESHIRE-CAT RABBIT HATTER)) returns the value (ALICE RABBIT HATTER). The CHESHIRE-CAT has disappeared—presumably his smile disappearing last.

Here is an example using these functions. Let's say we have previously set the value of A to be ALICE, R to be RABBIT, H to be HATTER, C to be CHESHIRE-CAT, and GUESTS to be the list (ALICE). Let's analyze what happens when we type in the expression below.

```
(APPEND GUESTS (REMOVE C (CONS R (LIST C)))).
```

Lisp always processes the most deeply nested expression—the one with the most parentheses—first. Reading the deepest expression (LIST C) first, Lisp returns the list (CHESHIRE-CAT). Then the CONS tacks RABBIT on the front to return the list (RABBIT CHESHIRE-CAT). Then the function REMOVE deletes CHESHIRE-CAT from the list and returns the value (RABBIT). Then the APPEND glues together the list (ALICE) with the list (RABBIT) to return the list (ALICE RABBIT).

Let's leave Wonderland for Mathland for a minute to consider another example. What do you think the value of this expression is?

```
(EVAL (CONS 'PLUS (LIST 5 7)))
```

Well, (LIST 5 7) simply returns the list (5 7). The CONS glues on the atom PLUS on the front to return the list (PLUS 5 7). And the EVAL then EVALuates it to return the number 12.

HOW A LISP FUNCTION WORKS

Figure 2

COMPUTER	USER	COMMENTS
_	(SETQ X 3)	*We type this expression after the prompt "_".*
3		*Lisp returns 3.*
_	(SETQ Y 4)	
4		
_	X	
3		*The value of X is 3, as set above.*
_	Y	
4		
_	(PRINT X)	
3		*Lisp printed a 3 in response to the command PRINT.*
3		*Now Lisp prints 3 because that is the value returned by the function call (PRINT X).*
_	(PLUS (TIMES 2 3) (DIFFERENCE 9 4))	
11		*That is: (PLUS 6 5) returns 11.*

ASSIGNING VALUES TO ATOMS

Figure 3

COMPUTER	USER	COMMENTS
_	(SETQ X (PLUS 3 4))	*Here the expression (PLUS 3 4) is evaluated, so X is set to 7 and the SETQ function returns a 7.*
7		
_	(SETQ X '(PLUS 3 4))	*Here the value of X is set to be literally the list (PLUS 3 4), because '(PLUS 3 4) is quoted.*
(Plus 3 4)		

Predicates

Let's continue to build our Lisp vocabulary by looking at some special functions called predicates, which tell true from false.

There are two special atoms in Lisp: T and NIL. These correspond to true and false, and there are certain functions called predicates (explained below) that return either T or NIL. For example, you might want to answer the question, "Does the patient have disease X?" You would instruct the program that in order for the patient to have disease X, symptoms 1, 2, 3, and 4 must be present. The predicate "AND" in Lisp would search the list of symptoms and require that all four of them were present before it returns the answer, "yes, the patient has disease X."

Let's explore six common predicates.

ATOM returns T (true) if its argument is an atom (as opposed to a list). Otherwise it returns NIL. (ATOM 5) returns T because 5 (or any number, by definition) is an atom. (ATOM '(ALICE)) returns NIL, since (ALICE) is a list, not an atom. (ATOM 'ALICE) returns T, because ALICE is an atom. You can say that (ATOM 'ALICE) returns T, or that it has the value T, or that it is true; they all mean the same thing.

LISTP returns T (true) if its argument is a list, otherwise it returns NIL (false). So (LISTP '(ALICE HATTER)) returns T because '(ALICE HATTER) is a list.

NOT returns the inverse of the truth of its argument. (NOT T) returns NIL. (NOT NIL) returns T. Earlier we saw that (ATOM 5) returns T because 5 is an atom. (NOT (ATOM 5)) returns NIL. Lisp first evaluates (ATOM 5) as true because 5 is an atom. It then evaluates (NOT T) and returns the opposite of true which is NIL.

AND returns T if *all* its arguments have the value T. In other words, if any argument evaluates to NIL, AND returns NIL. (AND (ATOM 'ALICE) T) will return T. (AND T NIL T) returns NIL because the three arguments "T", "NIL", and "T" are not all true. (AND T (NOT (ATOM 5))) returns NIL because (NOT (ATOM 5)) is NIL.

OR returns T if *any* of its arguments have the value T. (OR NIL T NIL) returns T. (OR (ATOM 'ALICE) NIL) returns T because ALICE is an atom. (OR NIL NIL NIL) returns NIL because none of its arguments is true.

EQUAL returns T if both of its arguments have equal values. Thus, (EQUAL 5 5) returns T. (EQUAL NIL 77) is NIL since NIL and 77 have different values. (EQUAL NIL NIL) is T. (EQUAL (PLUS 5 3) 8) also returns T. (EQUAL (ATOM 'ALICE) (ATOM 5)) returns T because ALICE and 5 are both atoms.

Properties of Atoms

In addition to assigning values to atoms, users can also assign "properties" to them. What is a property? Consider the lowly lemon. Its "color" property is yellow, its "taste" property is sour, and its "size" property is small. To store these properties in association with the atom LEMON, we can put the following list on LEMON's "property list": (COLOR YELLOW TASTE SOUR SIZE SMALL).

The function PUTPROP assigns properties to an atom's property list. (PUTPROP 'LEMON 'COLOR 'YELLOW) puts the COLOR property with its value YELLOW on the property list of LEMON. Note that the order of the arguments in PUTPROP is important. The first argument is the atom to be given the property. The second is the name of the property, and the third is the value of the property.

GETPROP fetches the value of a property. (GETPROP 'LEMON 'COLOR) will return the value YELLOW. See if you can figure out what is happening in the following expression:

```
(PUTPROPR 'PEAR 'COLOR (GETPROP 'LEMON
'COLOR))
```

First the GETPROP function returns the value YELLOW. Then the PUTPROP function puts this value onto the COLOR property of PEAR.

Property lists can be used to store lots of information in association with an atom. Earlier we showed a medical property list: (AGE 32 SEX FEMALE RACE CAUSASIAN CHIEF-COMPLAINT NAUSEA DX PREGNANT). These could be created by a series of PUTPROP commands: (PUTPROP 'PATIENT-1 'AGE 32), (PUTPROP 'PATIENT-1 'SEX 'FEMALE), etc. (There is another command, SETPROPLIST, which allows you to assign a list of properties more efficiently than repeating PUTPROP each time.)

UNLIKE MANY LANGUAGES, LISP DOES NOT RESTRICT THE VALUES OF ITS VARIABLES TO A SPECIFIC KIND OF DATA.

Once this list is completed, PATIENT-1 has the properties AGE, SEX, RACE, CHIEF-COMPLAINT, and DX. The values of these properties for PATIENT-1 are 32, FEMALE, CAUCASIAN, NAUSEA, and PREGNANT.

Here's how we might increase the patient's age by one year (PUTPROP 'PATIENT-1 'AGE (PLUS 1 (GETPROP 'PATIENT-1 'AGE))). The Lisp program prints 33 because this is the value returned by the PUTPROP.

Here's how we give our patient several diagnoses:

(PUTPROP 'PATIENT-1 'DX '(PREGNANT HYPERTENSION HYPERTHYROID)). Now let's remove a diagnosis from the list and have Lisp print the resulting list:

```
(PRINT (PUTPROP 'PATIENT-1 'DX (REMOVE
                'HYPERTENSION (GETPROP
                'PATIENT-1 'DX))))
(PREGNANT HYPERTHYROID)
```

Conditional Expressions: COND and IF

The function COND is Lisp's version of the familiar "*if-then-else*" expression found in most high level languages. A typical *if-then-else* statement might be: "If today is a weekday then go to work, else (if it is not a weekday) sleep in." The equivalent COND clause in Lisp would be:

```
(COND ((TODAY IS A WEEKDAY) (GO TO WORK))
      ((TODAY IS NOT A WEEKDAY) (SLEEP IN)))
```

The syntax of a COND clause looks like the following example:

```
(COND (A B)
      (C D)
      (E F)
      ....)
```

A, B, C, etc., can each be atoms or function calls. A COND works like this: If A is true, return the value of B; else, if C is true, return the value of D; else, if E is true, return the value of F, and so on. A COND expression, like every other list in Lisp, returns something. It returns the value of the clause that succeeded. If none of the clauses are true, it returns NIL.

For example, suppose we have previously written (SETQ PERSON 'ALICE), so the value of PERSON is ALICE. Now suppose we want to check to see who is a person and who is not:

```
(COND ( (EQUAL PERSON 'HATTER) (PRINT (LIST
        'REJECT PERSON) ))
      ( (EQUAL PERSON 'ALICE) (PRINT (LIST
        'ACCEPT PERSON) )))
```

The COND first checks to see if PERSON is equal to HATTER. It isn't, so the program checks to see if PERSON equals ALICE. It is, so the program executes the last expression and prints (ACCEPT ALICE). The COND expression itself returns this list as its value: (ACCEPT ALICE). Note that it does not return the *text* of the second argument "PRINT (LIST 'ACCEPT PERSON)". It returns the *value* of this argument, which is "ACCEPT ALICE."

Moving from Wonderland to Healthland, let's consider the following little *if-then* rule:

If Polycystic-Kidney = T
then Renal-Abnormality = T

This rule could be written in the COND form as follows:

```
(COND
( (EQUAL POLYCYSTIC-KIDNEY T) (SETQ RENAL-
ABNORMALITY T) ) )
```

In many artificial intelligence systems, the rules used for inference are represented with this COND structure. The "if" part is the premise, and the "then" part is the action or conclusion. Such rules usually do not have an "else" part. The "else" is handled by other rules.

THE GOLDEN RULE OF ARTIFICIAL INTELLIGENCE

The Golden Rule of artificial intelligence is to separate domain knowledge from the inference engine. Domain knowledge is a collection of facts and rules about a *subject*. For example, medical domain knowledge is a collection of facts and rules about diseases, symptoms, drugs, and so on. The inference engine is a program or set of rules of *logic* that allow you to reach conclusions using the facts and rules of the domain. In mathematics, for example, the inference engine is the set of rules concerning addition, multiplication, division, etc. The mathematical inference engine says that 2 + 2 = 4 is a correct conclusion; 2 + 2 = 5 is incorrect. The same inference engine applies to all numbers you may wish to add.

The rules of formal mathematical logic are often used to make an inference engine in expert systems and other artificial intelligence programs. In fact, one definition of an inference engine is that it is independent and can be transported from program to program. In our sample expert system, Minimycin, which will appear in a later issue of *M.D. COMPUTING*, we put the domain knowledge (facts and rules about medicine) into property lists, and we use a "rule interpreter" to manipulate this set of knowledge. We store the premise and action of rules on property lists so that they can be stored in a knowledge base separate from the program.

Let's construct a rule called RULE-1. First we store the premise (fact) of RULE-1:

```
(PUTPROP 'RULE-1 'PREMISE '(AND (EQUAL SEX
                                 'FEMALE)
                                (EQUAL AGE
                                 'ADULT)
                                (EQUAL
                                 SYMPTOM
                                 'DYSURIA)))
```

NESTING LISP EXPRESSIONS

Figure 4

COMPUTER	USER	COMMENTS
-	(SETQ X '(PLUS 3 4))	*Lisp sets X to be literally (PLUS 3 4) because of the quote mark.*
(PLUS 3 4)		
-	X	
(PLUS 3 4)		*Lisp types the value of X.*
-	(PLUS 5 (EVAL X))	
12		*Lisp EVALuates the value of X—which is (PLUS 3 4)—to get the value 7, then adds it to 5.*

Then we store the action of RULE-1, like this:

```
(PUTPROP 'RULE-1 'ACTION '(SETQ ORGANISM
'E.COLI))
```

Instead of having the medical knowledge hidden in a massive computer program, we can easily find and (with some practice) read it. All our knowledge will be stored on property lists of atoms like RULE-1. But how can we use this stored knowledge to make decisions? Our old friend EVAL (one of Lisp's principal features) helps us out.

Evaluating a Rule

The function EVAL is used to evaluate rules. First let's review how EVAL works on the sample we saw in Figure 4.

The function EVAL lets us evaluate X an additional time. The first time we get the value of X as (PLUS 3 4). We then EVALuate this value and get 7.

Here's another example of EVAL:

Computer	User
-	(SETQ A 'B)
B	
-	(SETQ B 'C)
C	
-	(EVAL A)
C	

EVAL can be used to evaluate arbitrary list structures, allowing us to construct computer code "on the fly." Our existing code can be used to construct more computer code, and then EVAL can execute it. In a sense, we let the computer program itself—proving that whoever said "computers can't program themselves" was wrong. Consider this example:

```
(SETQ OPERATION (COND ((EQUAL DAY
                       'MONDAY) 'TIMES)
                      ((EQUAL DAY
                       'TUESDAY) 'PLUS)))
(EVAL (LIST OPERATION 2 3))
```

On Mondays the EVAL will return 6, and on Tuesdays it will return 5.

We use EVAL to evaluate properties retrieved from property lists. Suppose we have previously set the PREMISE and ACTION properties of RULE-1 just as above. The (GETPROP 'RULE-1 'PREMISE) returns:

```
(AND (EQUAL SEX 'FEMALE)
     (EQUAL AGE 'ADULT)
     (EQUAL SYMPTOM 'DYSURIA))
```

Let's also suppose we have previously set the values of SEX, AGE, and SYMPTOM to be FEMALE, ADULT, and DYSURIA. Then, if we enter the following list, we can evaluate the premise of a rule:

```
(EVAL (GETPROP 'RULE-1 'PREMISE))
```

The EVAL evaluates our rule's premise and returns T because each of its clauses is true.

In a rule-based expert system, we want to evaluate rules often, so it makes sense to define a new function, EVALUATE-RULE, to do this. EVALUATE-RULE should act as follows:

If
  the premise of the rule is true,
Then
  evaluate the action of the rule.

Here is the Lisp definition of EVALUATE-RULE:

```
(DEFINE '((EVALUATE-RULE (RULE)
          (COND
            ((EVAL (GETPROP RULE 'PREMISE))
             (EVAL (GETPROP RULE 'ACTION)
```

EVALUATE-RULE first gets the PREMISE of RULE and EVALuates it. If the premise is true, the ACTION of RULE is retrieved and EVALuated.

ITERATION AND RECURSION CONTROL PROGRAMS

We are almost ready to describe how a miniature expert system works. Before proceeding, we need to explain the control of Lisp programs. Two commonly used techniques in all computer languages are iteration and recursion. Iteration means "do something repeatedly" and is accomplished with the "FOR . . . NEXT" loop in BASIC, or the "DO" loop in FORTRAN. In Lisp, when you want to do a series of things, you generally give it a list of things and tell it to do them. To signal Lisp of your intention, you put the atom PROG, short for program, at the front of the list. For example, let's define a program that repeatedly prints numbers:

```
(DEFINE '((PRINT-NUMBERS ()
          (PROG ()
             (PRINT 1)
             (PRINT 2)
             (PRINT 3)
             (PRINT 4)))))
```

When you call PRINT-NUMBERS, it will print 1 2 3 4. However, suppose you want to print all the numbers up to some arbitrary number N. To do this it would be easier to use iteration:

```
(DEFINE'((PRINT-NUMBERS (N)
          (PROG ()
             (FOR NUMBER FROM 1 TO N DO
                (PRINT NUMBER))))))
```

Then, (PRINT-NUMBERS 6) would produce 1 2 3 4 5 6. The expression (FOR NUMBER FROM 1 TO N DO . . .) makes Lisp loop, or iterate, and print NUMBER with the values from 1 to N. This syntax is very un-Lispish, but many dialects of Lisp allow it anyway to make it easier for the user to write programs in the form most familiar to programmers.

Another way to control programs is by using recursion. A recursive function calls itself repeatedly, like an image repeating itself endlessly in two facing mirrors. In the coming Minimycin article you will see a function "FIND-VALUE," which is recursive. FIND-VALUE tries to find the value of a variable. However, to do this, it sometimes has to find the value of some other variable first. So FIND-VALUE will call FIND-VALUE to find the value of that other variable. Because FIND-VALUE calls itself, it is a recursive function.

If you wanted to print an infinite string of numbers (not recommended because it takes too long), you could use recursion:

```
(DEFINE '((PRINT-NUMBERS (N)
          (PROG ()
             (PRINT N)
             (PRINT-NUMBERS (PLUS N 1))))))
```

(PRINT-NUMBERS 4) would start printing 4 5 6 7 8 9 . . . and would keep going until your system stopped or you forced Lisp to break. In this example, PRINT-NUMBERS is recursive because it first prints the value of its argument (N), and then calls itself with a new argument of N plus 1. As written, this is a bad function because it never stops. It is an "infinite loop." The programmer must be sure to include some command or

LISP FUNCTIONS

For each reference, here are brief definitions of the Lisp functions described in the article. All functions have the form: (function-name argument-1 argument-2 ... argument-n).

Remember, in Lisp, NIL = False and T = True. Anything other than NIL is also considered to be True.

(AND V W ... Z)	*Returns T if all of V, W, ... Z are true.*
(APPEND LIS1 LIS2)	*Makes a new list by gluing together the lists LIS1 and LIS2.*
(ATOM X)	*Returns T if X is an atom.*
(COND (A B) (C D))	*Lisp's version of if-then-else. If A then B, else if C then D.*
(CONS ATM LIS)	*Inserts the atom ATM at the front of the list LIS.*
(DIFFERENCE N M)	*N minus M.*
(EQUAL X Y)	*Returns T if X and Y are equal.*
(EVAL X)	*Forces a second evaluation of X. (Lisp automatically evaluates X once.)*
(GETPROP ATM PROP)	*Gets the value of the property PROP for the atom ATM.*
(LIST V W X ... Z)	*Returns its arguments collected into one list.*
(LISTP X)	*Returns T if X is a list.*
(NOT X)	*Returns the logical inverse of X.*
(OR V W X ... Z)	*Returns T if any of V, W, X, ... Z is T.*
(PLUS M N)	*M + N*
(PRINT X)	*Prints the value of X at the terminal.*
(PUTPROP ATM PROP VAL)	*Puts the property PROP on the property list of ATM with the value VAL.*
(REMOVE ATM LIS)	*Removes the atom ATM from the list LIS.*
(SETQ X Y)	*Sets X to the value of Y.*

logical control which tells the program to stop.

Onward to Minimycin

This wraps up our tutorial. If you understood most of this, then you should be able to understand the Lisp code of the Minimycin program easily. Just reading examples, it is sometimes difficult to understand a language. Being able to experiment is tremendously helpful. You'll learn Lisp a lot better if you can work with it on a computer.

A note on Lisp dialects

Several different versions of Lisp are available for microcomputers. These include TLC Lisp for Z-80 computers under CP/M and Apple II's, from The Lisp Company of Los Gatos, California; muLisp for the Intel 8080, 8085, and Z80-based computer under CP/M, from Microsoft; APP-L-LISP for the Apple II, from Datasoft in Los Angeles; IQ-Lisp for the IBM PC, from Integral Quality of Seattle; and Lisp for the TRS-80, from Supersoft of Champaign, Illinois. Any of these Lisps should be suitable for running Minimycin, although some may require slight changes in syntax. □

REFERENCES

If this article whets your appetite for learning Lisp, there are a few good primers that you may want to get. As a next step after this article, the Gloess book is an inexpensive guide. The textbooks by Siklossy and Winston & Horn provide more comprehensive coverage.

Gloess PY. Understanding Lisp: a concise introduction to the language of artificial intelligence. Sherman Oaks, CA: Alfred Publishing, 1982.

Siklossy L. Let's talk Lisp. Englewood Cliffs, NJ: Prentice-Hall, 1980.

Teitleman W. INTERLISP reference manual. Palo Alto, CA: Xerox Palo Alto Research Center, 1978.

Winston PH, Horn BKP. LISP. Reading, MA: Addison-Wesley, 1981.

MINIMYCIN: A MINIATURE RULE-BASED SYSTEM

MICHAEL G. WALKER, ROBERT L. BLUM, M.D., Ph.D., AND LAWRENCE M. FAGAN, M.D., Ph.D.

Artificial intelligence (AI) systems, in which computers perform tasks that would show intelligence if performed by a human, are already in frequent clinical use in a number of hospitals [1–2, 7]. Articles on artificial intelligence have appeared in the *New England Journal of Medicine* [3] and the *Journal of the American Medical Association* [4]. (Good collections on AI and medicine include [5] and [6].)

Existing expert systems have attempted to diagnose [3] and recommend therapy [2, 4], teach medical students [5], plan genetic engineering experiments, monitor patients in intensive care units [1, 7], advise about oncology protocols [2], and automate the discovery of new knowledge from medical databases [8]. As a branch of computer science, however, artificial intelligence is far larger than the field of expert systems. It also involves such tasks as understanding written and spoken English, robotics, and computer vision.

ROBERT L. BLUM, M.D., Ph.D.
Robert Blum is principal investigator of the RADIX Project in the Stanford Computer Science Department. The goal of RADIX is the automated discovery and confirmation of medical knowledge from large clinical databases. He received his B.S. in mathematics from the Massachusetts Institute of Technology in 1969, and his M.D. from the University of California Medical School at San Francisco in 1973. From 1976 to 1979 he was a postdoctoral fellow in the Stanford University Division of Clinical Pharmacology. He received his Ph.D. in computer science and biostatistics from Stanford University in 1982.

MICHAEL G. WALKER
Michael Walker is a computer scientist with Hewlett-Packard Labs, involved in the development of knowledge-based systems. Prior to joining HP, he was on the staff of the Stanford University Computer Science Department, where he worked on the RADIX project for automated medical discovery.

LAWRENCE M. FAGAN, M.D., Ph.D.
Lawrence Fagan is a Senior Research Associate in the Department of Medicine at Stanford University, and Project Director for the ONCOCIN project, an expert system designed to aid in the therapy selection process for complicated cancer protocols. He received a B.S. in interdisciplinary science from the Massachusetts Institute of Technology in 1973, a Ph.D. in computer science from Stanford in 1980, and a M.D. degree from the University of Miami in 1983.

To understand the potential of AI systems in medicine, the physician needs an idea of how they work. Our intent in this article is to introduce an example of one type of artificial intelligence, the expert system, using a small program we built called *Minimycin.*

Minimycin was designed to illustrate some of the features of a subclass of expert systems called *rule-based* systems. The methods of rule-based systems are incorporated in almost all new systems. *Minimycin*, derived from the MYCIN and EMYCIN programs developed at Stanford University [9, 10] is a relatively simple program for teaching Lisp and principles of rule-based systems. A reading of our article "An Introduction to Lisp" (*M.D. COMPUTING,* Vol. 2, No. 1) will help you to understand *Minimycin.*

Our sample medical knowledge base, drawn from the domain of urinary tract infections, consists of only ten rules. While these rules are plausible, we would hate to think of anyone treating a urinary tract infection based on them. Some of the extensions that would be necessary to make *Minimycin* a practical system are noted later. The rule base used here is only for illustration.

The important artificial intelligence concepts that we hope you will learn about by studying *Minimycin* are:

- Rules as used in artificial intelligence;
- Rule chaining;
- Rule trees;
- Rule indexes;
- Using rules to infer the value of objects;
- Using property lists to store
  (*a*) the premise of a rule,
  (*b*) the conclusion of a rule,
  (*c*) the list of rules relevant to an object (rule index),
  (*d*) the values of objects.

RULES

In English, a rule about urinary tract infections might look like this:

If the patient is female, adult, and has dysuria,
then the identity of the organism is E. Coli.

This same rule, translated into the language of this program, would appear this way:

```
If     (AND    (FIND-VALUE 'FEMALE)
               (FIND-VALUE 'ADULT)
               (FIND-VALUE 'DYSURIA))
  Then (ASSERT  'IDENTITY   'E. COLI)
```

The knowledge base for this urinary tract infection example is quite small; it contains only ten rules. Here are the rules in the knowledge base:

R1 If the patient has a urinary tract infection and abnormal urologic anatomy,
then conclude that the identity of the urinary organism is enterococcus.

```
If    (AND (FIND-VALUE 'URINARY-TRACT-
             INFECTION)
           (FIND-VALUE 'ABNORMAL-
             UROLOGIC-ANATOMY))
 Then (ASSERT 'IDENTITY 'ENTEROCOCCUS)
```

R2 If the patient has had urologic manipulation,
then conclude that abnormal urologic anatomy is true.

```
If    (FIND-VALUE 'UROLOGIC-
        MANIPULATION)
 Then (ASSERT 'ABNORMAL-UROLOGIC-
        ANATOMY T)
```

FUNCTIONS IN MINIMYCIN

The functions used in *Minimycin* are

ASKYESNO, ASSERT, CREATE-RULE-INDEX, EVALUATE-RULE, FIND-VALUE, INITIALIZE-MINIMYCIN, PRINT-VALUES, READ-RULE-ACTION

The definition of each of these functions is given below. (Note that a square bracket at the end of an expression may represent any number of end parentheses.)

```
(ASKYESNO
  [LAMBDA (STRING)
          (* ASKYESNO prompts the user to answer YES or NO in
          response to the prompt STRING. ASKYESNO stays in a
          DO loop until either YES or NO is entered.)
     (PROG (VALUE ANSWERED)
          (PRIN1 STRING)
          (PRINT (QUOTE :))
          (TERPRI)
          [until ANSWERED
             do (PROG NIL
                      (SETQ VALUE (READ))
                      (SETQ VALUE (SELECTQ VALUE
                                     ((YES Y y yes)
                                      (SETQ ANSWERED T)T)
                                     ((NO N n no)
                                      (SETQ ANSWERED T) NIL)
                                     (PROG NIL
                                           (PRINT
                                            "Enter either Y or N"]
          (RETURN VALUE])
 (ASSERT
  [LAMBDA (ATTRIBUTE NEW-VALUE)
          (*ASSERT puts the value stated in the action of a
          rule on the VALUE property of the attribute.)
     (PROG (PREVIOUS-VALUE)
          (SETQ PREVIOUS-VALUE (GETPROP ATTRIBUTE (QUOTE VALUE)))
          [SETQ NEW-VALUE (COND
             ((NULL PREVIOUS-VALUE)
              NEW-VALUE)
             ((ATOM PREVIOUS-VALUE)
              (LIST NEW-VALUE PREVIOUS-VALUE))
             ((LISTP PREVIOUS-VALUE)
              (CONS NEW-VALUE PREVIOUS-VALUE]
          (RETURN (PUTPROP ATTRIBUTE (QUOTE VALUE)
                           NEW-VALUE])
(CREATE-RULE-INDEX
  [LAMBDA NIL
          (* CREATE-RULE-INDEX creates the rule
          index. This is done by putting the list of
          relevant rules on the property list of each
          attribute.)
          (for ATTRIBUTE in ATTRIBUTES
             do (for RULE in ALL-RULES
                  do (COND
                     ((EQ (CADAR (GETPROP RULE (QUOTE ACTION)))
                          ATTRIBUTE)
```

```
            (PUTPROP ATTRIBUTE (QUOTE RELEVANT-RULES)
                     (CONS RULE (GETPROP ATTRIBUTE
                                         QUOTE RELEVANT-RULES])

(EVALUATE-RULE
  [LAMBDA (RULE)
          (* EVALUATE-RULE gets the premise of a rule and
          evaluates it. If it is true, it gets the action
          and evaluates it.)
     (COND
       ((EVAL (GETPROP RULE (QUOTE PREMISE)))
         (EVAL (GETPROP RULE (QUOTE ACTION])

(FIND-VALUE
  [LAMBDA (ATTRIBUTE)
          (* FIND-VALUE is the top-level function in
          Minimycin. It is explained in detail in the text.)
     (PROG (CONCLUSIONS)
          (RETURN (COND
                    ((SETQ CONCLUSIONS (GETPROP ATTRIBUTE (QUOTE VALUE)))
                      CONCLUSIONS)
                    ((SETQ RULELIST (GETPROP ATTRIBUTE (QUOTE RELEVANT-RULES)))
                      [for RULE IN RULELIST do (EVALUATE-RULE RULE)
                         unless (MEMBER (READ-RULE-ACTION RULE)
                                        (GETPROP ATTRIBUTE (QUOTE VALUE]
                      (GETPROP ATTRIBUTE (QUOTE VALUE)))
                    (T (PUTPROP ATTRIBUTE (QUOTE VALUE)
                                (ASKYESNO ATTRIBUTE])

(INITIALIZE-MINIMYCIN
  [LAMBDA NIL
          (* INITIALIZE-MINIMYCIN initiates the property
          lists of the attributes and creates the rule index
          needed to run Minimycin.)
     (PROG NIL
          (for ATTRIBUTE in ATTRIBUTES do (PUTPROP ATTRIBUTE
                                                   (QUOTE VALUE)
                                                   NIL))
          (for ATTRIBUTE in ATTRIBUTES do (PUTPROP ATTRIBUTE
                                                   (QUOTE
                                                     RELEVANT-RULES)
                                                   NIL))
          (CREATE-RULE-INDEX])

(PRINT-VALUES
  [LAMBDA (PROPERTY)
          (* PRINT-VALUES prints either the VALUES or the
          RELEVANT-RULES for all the attributes as indicated
          by PROPERTY. The default is VALUE.)
     (PROG NIL
          (for ATTRIBUTE in ATTRIBUTES
             do (PRINT (LIST ATTRIBUTE (GETPROP ATTRIBUTE
                                                (COND
                                                  (PROPERTY)
                                                  (T (QUOTE VALUE])

(READ-RULE-ACTION
  [LAMBDA (RULE)
          (* This function gets the VALUE to be deduced for an
          ATTRIBUTE by a rule. CADDR gets the third element in
          the list.)
     (CADDR (GETPROP RULE (QUOTE ACTION])
```

R3 If the patient has had catheterization or cystoscopy, then conclude that urologic manipulation is true.

```
If   (OR (FIND-VALUE 'CATHETERIZATION)
         (FIND-VALUE 'CYSTOSCOPY))
Then (ASSERT 'UROLOGIC-MANIPULATION T)
```

R4 If the patient has a renal abnormality, then conclude that abnormal urologic anatomy is true.

```
If   (FIND-VALUE 'RENAL-ABNORMALITY)
Then (ASSERT 'ABNORMAL-UROLOGIC-
       ANATOMY T)
```

R5 If the patient has polycystic kidneys, then conclude that renal abnormality is true.

```
If   (FIND-VALUE POLYCYSTIC-KIDNEYS)
Then (ASSERT 'RENAL-ABNORMALITY T)
```

R6 If the patient is female, adult, and has dysuria, then conclude that the identity of the urinary organism is E. coli.

```
If   (AND (FIND-VALUE 'FEMALE)
          (FIND-VALUE 'ADULT)
          (FIND-VALUE 'DYSURIA))
Then (ASSERT 'IDENTITY 'E. COLI)
```

R7 If the patient is immunosuppressed and has mycelia in the urine, then conclude that the urinary organism is a fungus.

```
If   (AND (FIND-VALUE
           'IMMUNOSUPPRESSED-HOST)
          (FIND-VALUE 'MYCELIA-IN-
           URINE))
Then (ASSERT 'IDENTITY 'FUNGUS)
```

R8 If the patient is receiving cancer chemotherapy or chronic steroids, then conclude that he is immunosuppressed.

```
If   (OR (FIND-VALUE CANCER-
          CHEMOTHERAPY)
         (FIND-VALUE CHRONIC-STEROIDS))
Then (ASSERT 'IMMUNOSUPPRESSED-HOST
       T)
```

R9 If the patient has a urinary tract infection, sterile urine culture, and disseminated TB, then conclude that the urinary organism is tubercle bacillus.

```
If    (AND (FIND-VALUE 'URINARY-TRACT-
           INFECTION)
           (FIND-VALUE 'STERILE-URINE-
           CULTURE)
           (FIND-VALUE 'DISSEMINATED-
           TB))
Then (ASSERT 'IDENTITY 'TUBERCLE-
     BACILLUS)
```

R10 If the patient is an immunosuppressed host and has TB bacteremia,
then conclude that patient has disseminated TB.

```
If    (AND (FIND-VALUE
           'IMMUNOSUPPRESSED-HOST)
           (FIND-VALUE 'TB-BACTEREMIA))
Then (ASSERT 'DISSEMINATED-TB T)
```

Rule Chaining

You may have noticed that the conclusions of some rules are used in the premises of other rules:

R3 If *catheterization* or *cystoscopy* are true,
Then *urologic manipulation* is true.

R2 If *urologic manipulation* is true,
Then *abnormal urologic anatomy* is true.

R1 If *abnormal urologic anatomy* and *urinary tract infection* are true,
Then the identity of the organism is enterococcus.

This is called chaining, because the rules link together to form a chain of reasoning, as follows:

CYSTOSCOPY
→
implies UROLOGIC MANIPULATION
→
implies ABNORMAL UROLOGIC ANATOMY
→
implies ENTEROCOCCUS

The Rule Tree

In most rule-based expert systems, the set of rules implicitly defines a tree of connected inferences. The conclusions of rules lower in the tree are used in the premises of rules higher up. The rule tree for urinary tract infections is shown in Figure 1.

A MINIMYCIN RULE TREE

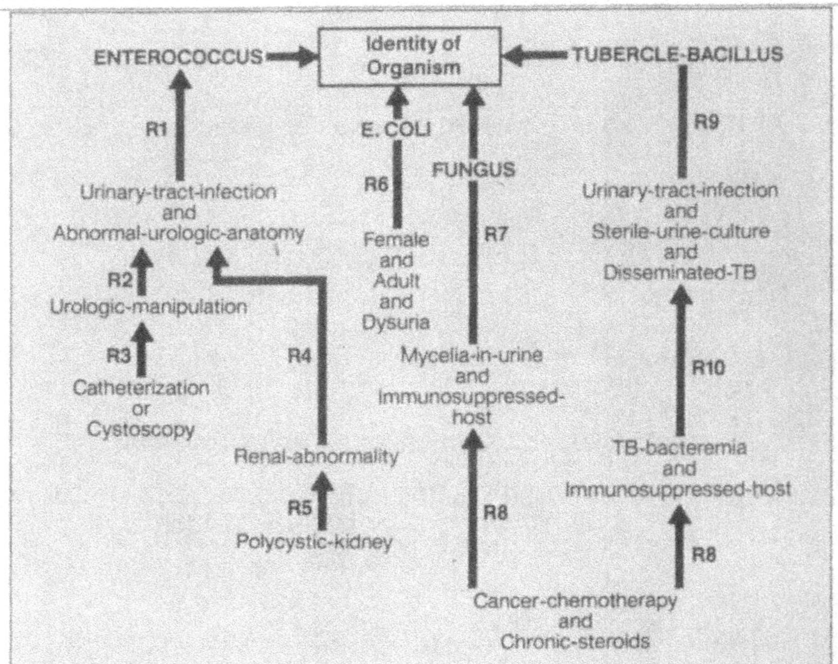

Figure 1.

To understand the way *Minimycin* works, examine the sample run shown as Figure 2; and then look at Figure 3, an example which shows the program's reasoning process in more detail.

GLOBAL VARIABLES

Minimycin uses two global variables: a list of all the rules called ALL-RULES, and a list of all the attributes called ATTRIBUTES.

```
(SETQ ALL-RULES '(R1 R2 R3 R4 R5 R6 R7 R8
    R9 R10))
(SETQ ATTRIBUTES '(ABNORMAL-UROLOGIC-
    ANATOMY ADULT CANCER-CHEMOTHERAPY
  CATHETERIZATION CHRONIC-STEROIDS
    CYSTOSCOPY DISSEMINATED-TB DYSURIA
  FEMALE IDENTITY IMMUNOSUPPRESSED-
    HOST MYCELIA-IN-URINE
  POLYCYSTIC-KIDNEY RENAL-
    ABNORMALITY STERILE-URINE-CULTURE
  TB-BACTEREMIA URINARY-TRACT-
    INFECTION)).
```

These lists are used by the *Minimycin* functions.

FUNCTIONS IN *MINIMYCIN*

The functions that perform back-chaining and rule evaluation constitute the core of *Minimycin*, and will be explained first. There are also functions for initializing the program and printing values that will be described later.

Back-Chaining and Rule Evaluation

The function FIND-VALUE is the central part of *Minimycin*. Its purpose is to find the value of the attributes of the program, however it can. The attributes are all the substantive entities of the rules: IDENTITY, IMMUNOSUPPRESSED-HOST, DYSURIA, CYSTOSCOPY, and so on. FIND-VALUE can find the value of these attributes in any of three ways. (The value of an attribute is stored on its VALUE property.)

- If the value has already been concluded by another rule, then FIND-VALUE returns that value.
- If the value is still unknown, then FIND-VALUE examines the RELEVANT-RULES property of the attribute. If the property is non-null, it means that there are rules that make conclusions about the attribute, and there-

A SAMPLE RUN OF MINIMYCIN

Figure 2. This is a sample run of *Minimycin.* The objective of the program is to find the identity of an infecting organism. (The user interaction is primitive because of the limited size of the program.) The program is started by typing (FIND-VALUE 'IDENTITY); it then prompts for the patient information it needs. The program moves downward through the tree.

EXAMPLE	COMMENTS
16_(INITIALIZE-MINIMYCIN) NIL	*{First, INITIALIZE-MINIMYCIN sets some variables and creates a rule index.}*
17_(FIND-VALUE 'IDENTITY)	*{FIND-VALUE tells the program to find the IDENTITY of the infecting organism.}*
URINARY-TRACT-INFECTION: Y CATHETERIZATION: N	*{The first rule concerned with IDENTITY is R1, which concerns urinary tract infections. The program asks the user if the patient has such an infection, and the user answers Yes.}*
CYSTOSCOPY: N	
POLYCYSTIC-KIDNEY: N	*{The program continues asking questions to gather patient information, traversing the rule tree, and the user responds Yes or No.}*
FEMALE: N	
MYCELIA-IN-URINE: N	
STERILE-URINE-CULTURE: Y	
CANCER-CHEMOTHERAPY: N	
CHRONIC-STEROIDS: Y	
TB-BACTEREMIA: Y	
TUBERCLE-BACILLUS	*{Minimycin concludes that the infecting organism is tubercle bacillus.}*

fore, FIND-VALUE will back-chain down this list of rules to try to find a value for the attribute. In doing this, it will try only those rules that make conclusions not already on the value list of the attribute. To do the back-chaining, it calls EVALUATE-RULE.

- As a last resort, if both of the above have failed, FIND-VALUE asks the user for the value of the attribute.

To interpret the rules that FIND-VALUE has found on the RELEVANT-RULES of the attribute, it calls EVALUATE-RULE, which first gets the code stored on the property list of the RULE under PREMISE and EVALuates it. If it is true, then it EVALs the ACTION of the RULE.

Suppose FIND-VALUE finds that it must invoke rules. Here's how it works. Say it is trying to find a value for IDENTITY. First, it gets the RELEVANT-RULES list from IDENTITY's property list. Second, it pulls the first rule off the front of the list (Rule R1). Then it calls EVALUATE-RULE on R1.

EVALUATE-RULE first gets the LISP code for the premise part of the rule from the rule's property list (here, from the property list of R1). It then evaluates the premise by calling EVAL on it. Next, if the premise evaluates as true, then EVALUATE-RULE gets the code for the action from the rule's property list and evaluates it.

The preceding paragraph conveys the essence of rule-based systems, the key reason that LISP is used to program rule-based systems. At the heart of *Minimycin* is this single idea:

```
(IF (EVAL (GETPROP RULE 'PREMISE))
 THEN (EVAL (GETPROP RULE 'ACTION))).
```

The EVAL in the premise causes the back-chaining. Before that premise is completely evaluated, hundreds of rules may need to be evaluated in a large production system.

The essence of LISP also lies in the two lines of code above. A piece of code, here the premise of the rule, is treated as a static data structure. When it is needed, it is "retrieved from memory," and then it is run as a program.

In executing the action of a rule, the function ASSERT is called. The essence of ASSERT is (PUTPROP ATTRIBUTE 'VALUE NEW-VALUE). In other words, its main function is to put the new value of the attribute stated by the action clause of the rule under the value part of the property list.

Initialization and Printing Values
The main function that looks after initialization is INITIALIZE-MINIMYCIN. It sets up the variables and calls CREATE-RULE-INDEX, which sets up the rule index, discussed in the next section.

The function PRINT-VALUES simply provides a convenient means for examining the property list of the attributes. For example, by calling (PRINT-VALUES 'RELEVANT-RULES), one can obtain a list of the attributes paired with a list of the rules that update each attribute. Simply calling (PRINT-VALUES) will print the values for each of the attributes for the last run of the program.

THE RULE INDEX

Suppose the system is trying to determine whether the patient

A MORE COMPLICATED CASE

Figure 3. This sample run includes a trace of the two vital functions in *Minimycin*: FIND-VALUE and ASSERT. Again, looking at the rule tree while we step through the program will help.

EXAMPLE	COMMENTS
26_(INITIALIZE-MINIMYCIN) NIL	*{First we initialize the program.}*
27_(FIND-VALUE 'IDENTITY) FIND-VALUE: ATTRIBUTE = IDENTITY	*{FIND-VALUE determines that the IDENTITY is not known. It retrieves the list of rules that conclude about IDENTITY (R1 R6 R7 R9). Each of these rules will be evaluated in turn.}*
FIND-VALUE: ATTRIBUTE = URINARY-TRACT-INFECTION	*{The premise of R1 contains the attribute URINARY-TRACT-INFECTION. FIND-VALUE is invoked to determine if URINARY-TRACT-INFECTION is true. No rules conclude about URINARY-TRACT-INFECTION, so it asks the user.}*
URINARY-TRACT-INFECTION: <u>Y</u> FIND-VALUE = T	*{The user indicates that the patient has a urinary tract infection. The value of (FIND-VALUE 'URINARY-TRACT-INFECTION) is T.}*
FIND-VALUE: ATTRIBUTE = ABNORMAL-UROLOGIC-ANATOMY	*{The program now knows that the patient has a urinary tract infection. However, to conclude that the patient has enterococcus, R1 requires that the patient also have abnormal urologic anatomy. FIND-VALUE is invoked on ABNORMAL-UROLOGIC-ANATOMY. It determines that the relevant rules are R2 and R4.}*
FIND-VALUE: ATTRIBUTE = UROLOGIC-MANIPULATION	*{R2 needs to know about UROLOGIC-MANIPULATION to conclude about ABNORMAL-UROLOGIC-ANATOMY. FIND-VALUE is invoked on UROLOGIC-MANIPULATION. The relevant rule is R3.}*
FIND-VALUE: ATTRIBUTE = CATHETERIZATION	*{R3 says, to conclude that the patient has had UROLOGIC-MANIPULATION, determine if CATHETERIZATION or CYSTOSCOPY have been done. FIND-VALUE is called. No rules conclude about CATHETERIZATION, so FIND-VALUE asks the user. The user answers <u>No</u>.}*

CATHETERIZATION: <u>N</u>
    FIND-VALUE = NIL
    FIND-VALUE:
    ATTRIBUTE = CYSTOSCOPY
	{CATHETERIZATION is false, so (FIND-VALUE 'CATHETERIZATION) is NIL. This means that the first part of the premise of R3 is false. Because the premise of R3 also looks for CYSTOSCOPY the user is asked if this is true.}

CYSTOSCOPY: <u>N</u>
    FIND-VALUE = NIL
  FIND-VALUE = NIL
	{The user answers <u>No</u>, so (FIND-VALUE 'CYSTOSCOPY) is NIL. Because neither CATHETERIZATION nor CYSTOSCOPY is true, R3 fails, and (FIND-VALUE 'UROLOGIC-MANIPULATION) is NIL and R2 fails.}

FIND-VALUE: ATTRIBUTE = RENAL-ABNORMALITY	*{The next rule relevant to ABNORMAL-UROLOGIC-ANATOMY is R4. R4 can use RENAL-ABNORMALITY to infer ABNORMAL-UROLOGIC-ANATOMY, so FIND-VALUE is invoked on RENAL-ABNORMALITY.}*
FIND-VALUE: ATTRIBUTE = POLYCYSTIC-KIDNEY	*{R5 uses POLYCYSTIC-KIDNEY to infer RENAL-ABNORMALITY. No rules infer POLYCYSTIC-KIDNEY, so FIND-VALUE asks the user.}*

POLYCYSTIC-KIDNEY: <u>Y</u>
      FIND-VALUE = T
      ASSERT:
      ATTRIBUTE = RENAL-ABNORMALITY
      NEW-VALUE = T
      ASSERT = T
	{The user answers <u>Yes</u>, so (FIND-VALUE 'POLYCYSTIC-KIDNEY) is true. The premise of R5 is true, so the action of R5 is executed (ASSERT 'RENAL-ABNORMALITY T).}

FIND-VALUE = T ASSERT:	*{Because (FIND-VALUE 'RENAL-ABNORMALITY) is true, the premise of R4 is true, and the action of R4 is executed (ASSERT 'ABNORMAL-UROLOGIC-ANATOMY T).}*

EXAMPLE	COMMENTS
ATTRIBUTE = ABNORMAL-UROLOGIC-ANATOMY NEW VALUE = T ASSERT = T FIND-VALUE = T ASSERT: ATTRIBUTE = IDENTITY NEW-VALUE = ENTEROCOCCUS	*{The program is continuing to search on this branch of the tree. Because both URINARY-TRACT-INFECTION and ABNORMAL-UROLOGIC-ANATOMY have been found to be true, the premise of R1 is true, and the action of R1 is executed (ASSERT 'IDENTITY 'ENTEROCOCCUS).}*
ASSERT = ENTEROCOCCUS	*{We have now been all the way down one branch of the tree and back up.}*
FIND-VALUE: ATTRIBUTE = FEMALE FEMALE: N FIND-VALUE = NIL	*{The next rule relevant to IDENTITY is R6. The premise of R6 contains the attribute FEMALE. (FIND-VALUE 'FEMALE) is invoked. No rule concludes about FEMALE, so the user is asked.} The user answers No. R6 cannot succeed, so no further questions are asked on this branch.}*
FIND-VALUE: ATTRIBUTE = MYCELIA-IN-URINE MYCELIA-IN-URINE: Y FIND-VALUE = T	*{The next rule concluding about IDENTITY is R7. R7's premise includes MYCELIA-IN-URINE. The user is asked, and answers Yes, so (FIND-VALUE 'MYCELIA-IN-URINE) is T.}*
FIND-VALUE: ATTRIBUTE = IMMUNOSUPPRESSED-HOST FIND-VALUE: ATTRIBUTE = CANCER-CHEMOTHERAPY	*{R7 also requires that IMMUNOSUPPRESSED-HOST be true, so FIND-VALUE is called.} {R8 use CANCER-CHEMOTHERAPY to conclude about IMMUNOSUPPRESSED-HOST. No rules apply, so the user is asked.}*
CANCER-CHEMOTHERAPY: N FIND-VALUE = NIL	*The user answers No, making (FIND-VALUE 'CANCER-CHEMOTHERAPY) be NIL. However, R8 can also use CHRONIC-STEROIDS.}*
FIND-VALUE: ATTRIBUTE = CHRONIC-STEROIDS CHRONIC-STEROIDS: Y FIND-VALUE = T	*{The user indicates that the patient is receiving CHRONIC-STEROIDS. R8 succeeds, so IMMUNOSUPPRESSED-HOST is true.}*
ASSERT: ATTRIBUTE = IMMUNOSUPPRESSED-HOST NEW-VALUE = T ASSERT = T FIND-VALUE = T ASSERT: ATTRIBUTE = IDENTITY NEW-VALUE = FUNGUS ASSERT = (FUNGUS ENTEROCOCCUS)	*{Both IMMUNOSUPPRESSED-HOST and MYCELIA-IN-URINE are true, so R7 succeeds, and asserts that the IDENTITY of the second organism is fungus. This is added to the previous finding of ENTEROCOCCUS.}*
FIND-VALUE: ATTRIBUTE = URINARY-TRACT-INFECTION FIND-VALUE = T	*{R9 is the final rule that concludes about IDENTITY. R9's premise includes URINARY-TRACT-INFECTION, but R1 already asked about it and the user answered Yes. This value was remembered, so (FIND-VALUE 'URINARY-TRACT-INFECTION) is true.}*
FIND-VALUE: ATTRIBUTE = STERILE-URINE-CULTURE	*{STERILE-URINE-CULTURE is also required for R-9, but the user indicates this is not true.}*
STERILE-URINE-CULTURE: N FIND-VALUE = NIL	
FIND-VALUE = (FUNGUS ENTEROCOCCUS) (FUNGUS ENTEROCOCCUS)	*{No further rules apply, so Minimycin concludes that the infecting organisms are FUNGUS and ENTEROCOCCUS.}*

has a RENAL-ABNORMALITY. It could be very slow to test every rule in a large system. One alternative is to keep a list of rules that make conclusions about RENAL-ABNORMALITY:

```
(PUTPROP 'RENAL-ABNORMALITY 'RELEVANT-
RULES '(R5))
```

In the current system only rule R5 concludes about renal abnormality.

The index is created once at the beginning of a consultation by the function CREATE-RULE-INDEX, which, in effect, does the following:

```
(PUTPROP 'IDENTITY 'RELEVANT-RULES '(R1 R6
  R7 R9))
(PUTPROP 'ABNORMAL-UROLOGIC-ANATOMY
  'RELEVANT-RULES '(R2 R4))
(PUTPROP 'RENAL-ABNORMALITY 'RELEVANT-
  RULES '(R5))
(PUTPROP 'UROLOGIC-MANIPULATION
  'RELEVANT-RULES '(R3))
(PUTPROP IMMUNOSUPPRESSED-HOST
  'RELEVANT-RULES '(R8))
(PUTPROP 'DISSEMINATED-TB 'RELEVANT-RULES
  '(R10))
```

For all the other attributes on the list ATTRIBUTES, the value stored under RELEVANT-RULES is NIL, because no rules are applicable.

POSSIBLE EXTENSIONS

Quite a number of extensions would be necessary to make this version of *Minimycin* a useful system. Here is a partial list:

- Improved user interface;
- Nonbinary attributes (instead of Y/N or T/NIL);
- Negative as well as positive conclusions (*is not* as well as *is*);
- Resolution of conflicting findings;
- A mechanism for handling uncertainty;
- Functions to provide explanations of the reasoning steps and to assist modification of the knowledge base.

ACKNOWLEDGMENTS

Our thanks to the MYCIN research group for creating the original *Mycin*. This paper was prepared using the facilities of SUMEX-AIM, a National Biotechnology Resource supported by the National Institutes of Health under grant number RR-00785. □

REFERENCES

1. Aikins JS, Kunz JC, Shortliffe EH, Fallat RJ. PUFF: an expert system for interpretation of pulmonary function data. Comp Biomed Res 1983; 16:199–208.

2. Shortliffe EH, Scott AC, Bischoff M, Campbell AB, van Melle W, Jacobs C. ONCOCIN: an expert system for oncology protocol management. Proceedings of the Seventh International Joint Conference on Artificial Intelligence, 1981:876–81.

3. Miller RA, Pople HE, Myers JD. INTERNIST-1: an experimental computer-based diagnostic consultant for general internal medicine. N Engl J Med 1982; 307:468–76.

4. Yu VL, Fagan LM, Wraith SM, Clancey WJ, Scott AC, Hannigan JF, Blum RL, Buchanan BG, Cohen SN. Antimicrobial selection by a computer: a blinded evaluation by infectious disease experts. JAMA 1979; 242:1279–82.

5. Clancey WJ, Shortliffe EH. Readings in artificial intelligence in medicine. Reading, MA: Addison-Wesley, 1984.

6. Szolovitz P, ed. Artificial intelligence in medicine (based on an American Association for the Advancement of Science symposium). Boulder, CO: Westview Press, 1982.

7. Weiss SM, Kulikowski CS, Galen RS. Developing microprocessor-based expert models for instrument interpretation. Proceedings of the Seventh International Joint Conference on Artificial Intelligence, 1981:853–5.

8. Blum RL. Discovery, confirmation, and incorporation of causal relationships from a large time-oriented clinical data base: the RX project. Comp Biomed Res 1982; 15:164–87.

9. Buchanan BG, Shortliffe EH. Rule-based expert systems: the MYCIN experiments of the Stanford heuristic programming project. Reading, MA: Addison-Wesley, 1984.

10. Shortliffe, EH. Computer based medical consultations: MYCIN. New York: Elsevier, 1976.

INDEX

Accumulators, 2, 3
ADA (language), 36, 100
Addition, *see* Binary arithmetic
Addresses, 3, 27–28
Aiken, Howard, 11
ALGOL, 31, 33, 34, 35–36, 87, 88, 92, 94
Algorithmic Language, *see* ALGOL
Altair 8800, 17
ALU, *see* Arithmetic logic unit
Amdek, 57
American Association of Medical Systems and Information (AAMSI), 83
American National Standards Institute (ANSI), 91
"Analytic Engine," 9, 11
APL (language), 89
Apple Computers, 54–55, 57, 81, 83, 86, 93, 95, 101
Applications, defined, 29
Arcnet, 110
Arithmetic logic unit (ALU), 2
Arrays, 33
Artificial intelligence, 127–128, 132, 135
Artificial Intelligence Corporation, 118
ASCII (American Standard Code for Information Interchange), 1, 25, 26, 79, 81, 84
  extended, 26
  use in bar coding, 73
Assembly language, 2, 13–14, 30–31, 32, 33, 87, 94, 95
  macro-assembly, 14
AT&T, 122, 124
Atari, 95, 101
Authoring and authoring systems, 38, 41–43

Babbage, Charles, 9, 11
Backup, 5, 6
Ballistic Research Laboratories, 11
Bar codes, 71–75
Bar graphs, 60
Baseband systems, 109
BASIC, 30, 31, 33, 35, 36, 73, 74–75, 88–91, 92, 94, 102
Baud rate, 5
  see also Data communications
Bell Laboratories, 11, 12, 123
Bell 212 modem, 80
BGS (graphics program), 65
Bidirectional logic, 5
Binary adder, 11
Binary arithmetic, 23–25
Binary digits, *see* Bits
Binary number systems, 9, 12
Bits, 1, 13, 23–28
  per second, *see* Baud rate
Block-structured languages, 36
Borland Systems, 93–94
BPS (graphics program), 67–69
Broadband systems, 109
Buffers, 5, 6–7, 81, 84
Bulletin board systems, *see* Remote Bulletin Systems
Burroughs, 94
Buses, 2, 23, 28
Bytes, 1, 27

C (language), 31, 33, 35, 36, 88, 91, 92, 94–96
Cables, in data communications, 77–78, 108, 111
CAI, *see* Computer-aided instruction
Card readers, 15
Cathode-ray tube (CRT), *see* Video-display tube
Central processing unit (CPU), 2–5, 6–7, 15, 16, 23, 27, 28
  use with programming languages, 30–31, 32
Character placement mode, 5
Christensen, Ward, 82
Clocks, 2, 5
CMOS, *see* Complementary metallic oxide semiconductors
Coaxial cables, 108, 111
COBOL, 14, 31, 34–35, 36, 87, 88, 94
Code 39, 72, 73
Color graphics boards, 58
Commodore, 122
Communications, *see* Data communications
Capatibility, 13
Compilers, 14, 88, 89, 90, 92, 93–94, 95–96, 103
Complementary metallic oxide semiconductors (CMOS), 5
CompuServe, 82–83, 86
Computer-aided instruction (CAI), 37–44
Computer-student interface, 42–43
Contention access, 110, 111
Continuous speech recognition, 48–50
Continuous variable-slope modulation, 45

Control bits, 7
Control Data Corporation, 37
Control language, *see* Job control language
Control unit (CU), 2
Controller, 6–7
Core memory, 3
  see also Random access memory
Cores, 3
Courseware, 38–44
  design and evaluation, 40–41
CPU, *see* Central processing unit
CP/M, 83, 101, 122
CRT (Cathode-ray tube), *see* Video-display tube
CU, *see* Control unit
Cursor, 16
Cyclic redundancy check (CRC), 82
Cylinders (on disks), 6

Data blocks, 6, 31
Data bus, 2
Data capture, 81
Data communication equipment (DCE), 78
Data communications, 77–86, 105–112
  errors, 82–83
  protocols, 107–108, 111, 112
  software, 80–82
  speed, 79–80
  troubleshooting, 85
  see also Local Area Networks
Data counter, 2, 3
Data exchange, between programs, 70
Data storage, 1, 6
Data structures
  in COBOL, 34–35
  in PASCAL, 92
Data termination equipment (DTE), 78
Data types, 32–33
Database management systems, 61, 88
Datagrams, 112
Datapoint (company), 110
dBase II, 88, 102, 103
Debuggers, 89
DEC (Digital Equipment Corporation), 16, 57, 86, 91, 110
Decimal arithmetic, 24
Defense Calculator, 12
Delaware, University of, 37, 39
Delivery-system software and hardware, 38–39
Digital Research, 91, 92, 100, 103, 122
Digitized speech, 45–46, 50
Direct access, *see* Random access
Direct memory access (DMA), 5
Discrete systems, 9
Discs, *see* Disks
Disks, 6, 15, 16
  formatting, 6
Display, *see* Video display
Division, *see* Binary arithmetic
DMA, *see* Direct memory access
Domain knowledge, 132
Dorlabs (company), 78
Dow Jones Information Service, 83
Draftsman (graphics program), 65, 67
Dumps, 14
Duplex, 78

EAPROM, *see* Electrically alterable programmable read only memory
EBCDIC (Extended Binary Coded Decimal Interchange Code), 1, 26, 79
Eckert, J. Presper, 11–12, 13
EDVAC (Electronic Discrete Variable Computer), 12
Electrically alterable programmable read only memory (EAPROM), 5
ENIAC (Electronic Numerical Integrater and Computer), 11
EPROM, *see* Erasable programmable read only memory
Erasable programmable read only memory (EPROM), 5
Ergonomics, in monitors, 57
Error checking/detection, 82, 103, 113
Ethernet, 110
Expert systems, 132–133, 135
Exponents, 27
External bus, 2, 6

Feature-based speech recognition, 49–50
Feedback, in computer-assisted instruction, 38
Fiberoptics, 108, 111
Files, 31
Fixed memory, *see* Read only memory
Floating point arithmetic, 27, 28
Floppy disks, 6, 15, 16, 31
Flow control
  in C, 94
  in data communications, 82
  in FORTRAN, 33–34
Formatting, *see* Disks
FORTH, 100
FORTRAN, 14, 30, 31–34, 36, 87, 88, 89, 90–91, 92, 103
  computations in, 33, 34
  use in computer-assisted instruction, 41, 43
Fractions, representation of, 26–27
Function keys, 16

Gas plasma monitors, 52–53
Gates, 3
General Electric, 94
GIRAPH, 64–65
GOTO statements, 33
Graphs and graphics, 58
  data entry, 61–62
  hard copy, 63–64
  labeling, 62
  programs, 59–70
  use in computer-assisted instruction, 40–41

Handshaking, 81–82, 84
Hard disks, 6
  see also Disks
Hardware, 15–16, 17, 23, 29
  defined, 13
Harvard University, 37
Hayes Smartmodem, 80, 84, 86
Hercules boards, 51, 58
Hewlett-Packard, 91, 100
Hexadecimal system, 28
High-order languages (HOL), 14, 15, 25, 27
Histograms, 60
Hitachi, 57
HOL, *see* High-order languages
Hollerith, Herman, 11
Honeywell, 94

IBM Corporation, 11, 12, 13, 57
IBM 360, 13
IBM 701, 12
IBM 7090, 12, 13
IBM-PC, 28, 30, 54–55, 57, 73, 81, 86, 93, 101, 102, 103
IC, *see* Integrated circuits
IF/THEN statements, 33–34
Illinois, University of, 37
Inference engines, 132
Input/output (I/O), 6–7, 16, 31
Instruction register, 2, 3
Integer format, 26
Integrated circuits (IC), 13
Integrated programs, 69–70
Intel Corporation, 17, 110
  8088, 28
Intellect (natural language system), 118
Interfaces, 5, 6–7
Interpreters, 88, 89, 90
I/O, *see* Input/output
Iteration, 133
Iverson, Kenneth, 100

Job control language (JCL), 14

Kay, Alan, 101
Kemeny, John, 88
Keyboards, 5, 6, 15–16
Kurtz, Thomas, 88
Kurzweil reader, 46

Large numbers, representation of, 26–27
Large-scale integration (LSI), 13
Leading bit, 25
Learning strategies, in computer-assisted instruction, 40–41
Leibniz, Gottfried Wilhelm von, 9
Libraries, defined, 34
LIFER, 117, 118
Line graphs, 61
Linear predictive coding (LPC), 45–46
Link loaders, 14
Liquid crystal displays (LCDs), 53
Lisa, 30, 101
  see also Apple Computers
LISP, 89, 100–101, 127–133
Local area networks (LAN), 105–114
  access, 110, 111
  protocol layers, 112
  reliability, 113
  services, 112
  single vs. multichannel systems, 109, 111
  user skills required, 113–114
  topology, 109–110, 111
LOGO, 101
LOL, *see* Low-order language
Lotus 1-2-3, 51, 102, 103
Low-order language (LOL), 31
  see also Assembly language
LPC, *see* Linear predictive coding
LSI, *see* Large-scale integration

Machine Intelligence Corporation, 118
Machine time, *see* Clocks
Macintosh, 30, 100, 101
  see also Apple Computers
Macros, 14, 102
Magnetic material, 6
  tape, 6, 12, 13, 14, 15, 16
Mark I, 11, 12
Mass storage, *see* Permanent storage
Massachusetts General Hospital, 37
  see also MUMPS
Mauchly, John, 11–12, 13
Menu systems, 119
MDM710, 83
MEDLINE, 48
Megahertz (MHz), defined, 2
Memory, *see* Working storage
Memory organization, 1–2, 16
Metallic oxide semiconductors (MOS), 3, 5
MHz, *see* Megahertz
Microde, 2
Microcomputers, 16, 17
Microsoft, 51, 73, 90, 91, 94, 102, 103, 122
  Word, 51
Minicomputers, 16–17
Minimycin, 135–142
Mnemonic instructions, 14, 30
MODEM-7, 82, 83, 84
Modems, 78–80, 84, 85, 86
Modula II, 100
Monitors, 5, 51–58
  characteristics, 53, 56–57
  selection, 57–58
MOS, *see* Metallic oxide semiconductors
Motorola 68000, 28
MS-DOS, 121, 122
MULTICS, 94
Multiplication, *see* Binary arithmetic
Multiprocessing, 15
Multiprogramming, 15, 16
MUMPS, 101–102, 124
MVS (operating system), 123, 125
MYCIN, 101, 135

N^2–N problem, 107–108, 113
Napier, John, 9
Natural language, 115–119
  in voice-activated systems, 50
  use in computer-assisted instruction, 43
  NEC (Nippon Electric Company), 57
  Net/One, 110, 112
  Network interface units (NIU), 108, 109–110, 112–113
  "New Pathways," 37
  Nonprocedural languages, 102

Oasis, 122
Ohio, University of, 37
On-the-job training, 39–40
Operating systems, 14, 15, 16, 25, 121–127
Oracle, 119
Overlays, 103

Paging, 28
Pappert, Seymour, 101
Parallel transmission, 6, 79
Parity bits, 1, 25–26, 79
Partitions, 16
PASCAL (languages), 31, 33, 35, 36, 88, 91–94, 103
Pascal, Blaise, 9
PBXs, 109
PC-TALK, 83
PDP series, 16
Peripheral devices, *see* Peripherals
Peripherals, 2, 5, 17
  interfacing with, 6
Permanent storage, 16, 30–31, 34–35
Phase I Systems, 122
Philco Corporation, 12
Photo equipment, in presentation graphics, 64
Pick (operating system), 121, 123
Pie charts, 60–61
PL/1 (language), 36, 99–100, 103
PLATO (Programmed Logic for Automated Teaching Operations), 37, 39
Plotters, 64, 66
Ports, *see* Input/output, RS232 ports
Predicates, 130–131
Princeton Graphics, 57
Printed circuits, 12–13
Printers, 5, 6, 15
  history, 12
  use in presentation graphics, 63–64
Process control, 16, 30
Processing cycles, 28
Programs
  counter, 2
  definition, 29
  storage, 27–28
Programmable read only memory (PROM), 5
Programming languages, 29–36, 87–104
PROM, *see* Programmable read only memory
Protocols, *see* Data communications
Pulse code modulation, in speech generation, 45
Punch cards, 11, 12

Quadram Corp, 57

Radio Shack, 83, 94, 95
Random access, 6, 15
Random access memory (RAM), 3, 6, 16, 23, 28
Read only memory (ROM), 2, 3, 5, 6, 16
Records, 31
Recursion, 94, 133
Registers, 2–4, 6, 23, 28, 30–31
Relays, 11, 12
Remington Rand, 12
Remote access, 15
Remote Bulletin Board Systems (RBBS), 83, 84, 86

Reverse polish notation (RPN), 100
ROM, *see* Read only memory
RS232 ports, 78, 79, 80, 83, 84
Rule-generated speech, 46, 50
Rules, 136–142
 chaining, 138–139
 evaluation, 132–133, 138–139
 index, 139–142

Sakata U.S.A. Corporation, 57
Sanyo, 57
Scaling, 26–27
SCAMP, 117–118
Scatter plot graphs, 61
Scientific notation, 26–27
Scientific programming, 32
Seattle, University of, 37
Secondary storage, *see* Permanent storage
Segment register, 28
Serial (sequential) access, 15
Serial transmission, 6, 78, 79
Servers, 107
Sign bit, 24–25
Silicon chips, 3, 5, 13
Slides, in presentation graphics, 63
Smalltalk, 101
SofTech Micorsystems, 93, 123
Software, 16, 17, 29
 definition, 13
 in communications, 80–86
Software Toolworks, 95, 101
Sony, 57
Source, The, 82, 86
Spaghetti code, 91
Speaker dependency, 48–50
Speech generation, 45–48, 50
 medical uses, 46–48
Speech recognition, 45, 48–50
Spreadsheet programs, 61–62
SRI International, 117
Status bits, *see* Control bits
Stibitz, George, 11
Stop bits, 79
Storage media, *see* Disks, Magnetic tape
Subroutines, 34, 91, 93
Subtraction, *see* Binary arithmetic
Symantec, 118
Symbolic assembly language, *see* Assembly language
System architecture, 15
Systems programs, 29, 94
 see also Operating systems
Sytek Corporation, 112

Tabulatory Machine Company, *see* IBM Corporation
Tape, *see* Magnetic tape
Telenet, 82, 86
Television sets, use as monitors, 57
Terminal emulation, 86
Texas Instruments, 17, 57, 118–119
3Com Corporation, 113
Time-sharing, 15
Token passing, 110, 111
Tracks, *see* Disks
Transistors (transfer resistors), 12, 13
Trinity Computing Systems, 107
Turbo-Pascal, 93–94, 102
Turtle graphics, 101
Tutoring, 41
Tymnet, 82

Ungermann-Bass, 110, 112
UNIVAC I (Universal Automatic Computer), 12
Universal Product Code (UPC), 72
UNIX, 94, 95, 103, 122, 123–125
USCD P-System, 93, 122
User communication, 31

Vacuum tubes, 11, 12
Vadic 3400, 80
Variable memory, *see* Random access memory
Variables, 30, 31, 33, 92, 129
VDT, *see* Video-display tube
Verification, *see* Parity
Very large scale integration (VLSI), 13
Video-display terminals, 5, 6, 16
 see also Monitors
Video-display tube (VDT), 15, 51
 see also Monitors
Video output, *see* Video display terminals
Virtual circuits, 112
Virtual memory, 28
VLSI, *see* Very large scale integration
VM (operating system), 123, 125
Voice output, *see* Speech generation
Voice recognition, *see* Speech recognition
von Neumann, John, 11–12, 13, 15
VT-100 (terminal), 86

Wang Corporation, 109
Whitesmith, 95
Winchester disks, *see* Hard disks
Wirth, Niklaus, 100
Word processing, 28, 51, 57–58, 61
Words, 30, 31
 defined, 2
 size, 2, 13, 23–28
Working storage (memory), 3–5, 6, 16, 30–31

Xerox, 101, 110

Zenith Data System Corporation, 57

www.ingramcontent.com/pod-product-compliance
Lightning Source LLC
Chambersburg PA
CBHW082006130926
51338CB00021B/50
* 9 7 8 1 4 6 1 2 8 3 2 1 8 *